Sirtfood Diet

Table of Contents

Introduction 1
Chapter 1: The Science of Sirtuins 2
Sirtuins Interaction with NAD+ 2
Sirtions are Proteins, So What? 3
History of Sirtuins 5
The Future of Sirtuins 7
Chapter 2: Sirtfood Diet and Aging 8
Weight Loss 8
Positive Influence on Genetics 9
Keeping Appetite Under Control 12
Preserve Muscle and Bone Mass 13
Blood Sugar Levels Under Control 14
Better Sleep 14
Fight Off Free Radicals 16
Reduced Stress and Anxieties 16
Anti-Aging Effects 17
Fight Chronic Diseases 18
Chapter 3: How to Get Started with the Sirtfood Diet When You're Over 50 20
Phase One 20
Phase Two 21
When to Stop 22
Chapter 4: Foods You Can Eat on the Sirtfood Diet 23
Chapter 5: How to Follow the Sirtfood Diet 25
Safety and Side Effects 26
Chapter 6: Sirtfoods for Life 28
Is Sirtfoods the New Superfoods? 29
Is it Healthy and Sustainable? 30
Summary 33
Breakfast Recipes 34
Cherry and Banana Smoothie 34
Banana and Green Smoothie 35
Breakfast Burrito 36

Chocolate Waffles 37

Pumpkin and Berries Quinoa 39

Chocolate, Peanut Butter and Chickpea Pancakes 40

Kale Wrapped Eggs...42

Artichoke Dip..43

Zucchini Noodles 45

Grapes and Green Tea Smoothie 46

Mango and Kale Smoothie...47

Pomegranate Smoothie...48

Zucchini and Blueberry Smoothie 49

Hot Pink Beet Smoothie 50

Vegetable Pancakes..51

Lunch Recipes...53

Lentil and Quinoa Salad 53

Ginger Brown Rice..54

Chickpea Salad..55

Kale Tacos...56

Chickpea and Avocado Salad 57

Spinach and Orange Salad.. 58

Roasted Tomatoes..59

Asparagus Soup 61

Roasted Brussel Sprouts 62

Green Bean Casserole 63

Kale Chips...65

Guacamole 66

Brussels Sprout Skewers..67

Quinoa Tacos 69

Ginger Veggie Stir-Fry 71

Dinner Recipes 73

Eggplant and Potatoes in Tomato Sauce 73

Lentil Vegetable Curry 74

Black Bean Stew..76

Vegetable Barley Soup 77

Sweet Potato and Corn Chowder 78

Pesto Broccoli Rice 80

Pea Soup 81

Lemon Basil Tofu 83

Pumpkin Soup 85

Broccoli Soup...86

Mushroom Steak 87

Pumpkin Chili..89

Wild Rice Mushroom Soup 91

Lentil with Spinach...93

Carrots and Quinoa Veggie Bowl.................................94

Dessert Recipes.. **96**

Chocolate and Avocado Pudding..................................96

Chocolate Covered Dates.. 97

Chocolate Chip Cookies..98

Pumpkin and Chocolate Brownies 100

Chocolate Bark 101

Strawberry and Banana Ice Cream............................ 102

No-Bake Chocolate Pie 103

Fudge Brownies... 104

Caramel Slice 106

Creamsicles... 108

No-Bake Cookies 109

Chocolate Strawberry Shake 110

Chocolate Clusters.. 111

Chocolate Pots 112

Maple and Tahini Fudge 113

Conclusion...**115**

Introduction

Similar to diet trends such as intermittent fasting and a plant-based diet, there is another rising star. The latest diet trend is called the Sirtfood diet. It is rapidly becoming a favorite diet among celebrities in Europe and is well-known for the fact that it allows chocolate and red wine.

Adele, among many other celebrities, says that the diet did wonders for their body and helped them lose a tremendous amount of weight in a short period. Now, you may be thinking that this is some sort of unsustainable health fad, and you are forgiven for thinking that. Attaching such a bold claim to a diet would raise more than a few eyebrows.

But as with many things in life, it's never that simple. Of course, you would lose a lot of weight quickly if you follow this diet, but it's not in the way that you think. It allows you to remain healthy and functional while shedding a lot of weight in the process.

This new diet is called the Sirtfood Diet. In this book, we will explore what the Sirtfood Diet really is, the science behind it, and the many ways you can incorporate this into your life.

Chapter 1: The Science of Sirtuins

To put it simply, Sirtuins helps to regulate your cell's health. As Sirtfood Diet relies on Sirtuins to do its magic, it is worth understanding in detail what Sirtuins can do for your body; but what is Sirtuins?

Sirtuins are a family of proteins. They help regulate your cells' health, and specifically, they play an important role in regulating cellular homeostasis or keeping the cell in balance. However, they only work when there is NAD+ in the system. NAD+ is Nicotinamide Adenine Dinucleotide, and it is a coenzyme present in all living cells.

Sirtuins Interaction with NAD+

Without going too much into the science mumbo jumbo, think of your body as an office populated by your cells. Every cell has a role to play in keeping you alive by being as efficient as possible, which is the ultimate goal. The cells also have their own personal goal, which is to remain ealthy and continue to work for as long and as efficiently as possible.

A company may change its priorities based on the market. To that end, someone needs to keep an eye on things. In a company, that would be the manager or the CEO who decides what gets done, who's going to do it, when the job needs to be done, and when a change of plan is needed.

Similarly, your body may change due to internal or external factors as well. The cells need to adapt to these changes to continue to achieve the ultimate goal. The manager or CEO here would be your sirtuins.

Sirtuins belong to a family of 7 proteins that play a crucial role in maintaining your cellular health. As mentioned before, they only work when there are NAD+ in the system. As enzymes, NAD+ is needed for your cell's metabolism as well as many other biological functions.

Going back to our office analogy, if the sirtuins are the CEO, then NAD+ is the company's finance. It pays the CEO, the water and electricity bills, and the office's rent. In short, the body wouldn't work without NAD+. The problem here is that the amount of NAD+ decreases with age, so sirtuins do not work as well as when you get older.

Sirtions are Proteins, So What?

As mentioned before, Sirtuins are a family of proteins, and if you may be thinking that these are dietary proteins found in foods such as beans, meats, and protein shakes, that's not it. In this case, we're talking about molecules called proteins, which have various functions within the cell.

One such example is hemoglobin, which is a member of the globin family of proteins. Hemoglobin helps get oxygen into your blood. The other half of the globin family is myoglobin, which distributes the oxygen into the cells, from the blood.

Overall, your body has almost 60,000 families of proteins. If you use the company analogy again, it will look like a multibillion-dollar company with countless departments and employees. Sirtuins work in one department with a specific function, whereas hemoglobin works in another department.

Three of the seven in the Sirtuins family work in the mitochondria, the powerhouse of the cell. Another three work in the nucleus. The last one works in the cytoplasm. They all work in the cell to ensure its optimal health. Although their roles are varied, their most primary role is to remove acetyl groups from other proteins.

Acetyl groups control certain reactions. They help proteins recognize other proteins and control how they will interact. So, if the proteins are the various departments of the cell and the DNA is the manager, then the acetyl groups are the availability status of the department.

For instance, sirtuin will check in with the acetyl of another protein to see if it is available. If so, sirtuin can work with that protein to make something happen, similar to how the CEO can work with another department to get something done.

Going back to sirtuins, they work with acetyl groups by doing "deacetylation." Simply put, they look for acetyl group on a molecule and then remove it, allowing the molecule to do its job.

So, one way that sirtuins work is to remove acetyl groups from biological proteins such as histones. For instance, sirtuins deacetylate histones, which are the proteins that are part of a condensed form of DNA called chromatin. The histone is a large and bulky protein that the DNA is wrapped around, similar to the light strands on a Christmas tree. When the histones contain an acetyl group, the chromatin is unwound or open.

When the chromatin is unwound, that means the DNA is being transcribed, which is an important process. But that does not mean that the chromatin must remain unwound as it is prone to damage in that position, just like how Christmas lights can get tangled or bulbs can be damaged if left on for too long.

So when the histones are deacetylated by sirtuins, the chromatin is tightly and neatly wound or closed so that gene expression is stopped or silenced, which helps prevent the DNA from being damaged.

Sirtuins seem to play a vital role in slowing down aging, and we have only known about them for 20 years. Their primary functions were discovered in the 90s. Ever since their discovery, many fascinated research flocked to study them, trying to understand their importance.

History of Sirtuins

It is only in the 90s did we start to understand their vital functions in the cells. However, their existence was discovered in the 70s by a geneticist Dr.

Amar Klar. He dubbed the first sirtuin SIR2 and identified it as a gene that allows yeast cells to mate.

Several years later, in the 90s, researchers discovered other homologous genes, or similar in structure, to SIR2 in many other living organisms such as worms and fruit flies. These SIR homologs are then dubbed sirtuins. Different living species have a different number of sirtuins. For instance, humans and mice have 7, yeast has five, and bacteria has one.

In 1991, Elysium co-founder and MIT biologist Leonard Guarente and a few graduate students such as Nick Austriaco and Brian Kennedy, conducted various experiments to gain a better understanding of how yeast age.

Purely by chance, Austriaco had attempted to cultivate many yeast strains from the samples he had kept in the fridge for many months. This was a stressful environment for the strains, and so many died off.

What was fascinating was the fact that the yeast strains that survived the ordeals have one thing in common. The strains that survived also lived the longest, even without subjecting them to the extreme environment. This was the start for Guarante to focus on these specific strains of yeast.

In time, SIR2 was discovered. It is a gene that promoted longevity in yeast. To this day, we still do not have enough evidence that this discovery can be extrapolated to humans. As such, more scientific studies need to be conducted on SIR2's effects on humans.

What is clear is that dramatically removing SIR2 reduced the lifespan of the yeast, and introducing more copies of SIR2 from one to two did the exact opposite. What we do not know is what activated SIR2 naturally.

Here is where acetyl groups come into the picture. At first, scientists thought that SIR2 could be a deacetylating enzyme, but no one knew if this was the case, considering that previous attempts to demonstrate such activity in a test tube did not yield any positive result. Guarante and his team, however, got as far as discovering that SIR2 in yeast could only deacetylate other proteins when there is NAD+ in the system.

So the research managed to yield a simple yet critical result. SIR2 does not do anything unless there is NAD+ in the system.

The Future of Sirtuins

There is so much we could learn from Sirtuins, and most of the scientific studies thus far have been on metabolic activities and aging. There are over 10,000 papers on sirtuins right now, and there may be some exciting discoveries in the future.

Chapter 2: Sirtfood Diet and Aging

As mentioned in the last chapter, there are various documents that prove the Sirtfood Diet could be effective. That said, if you are wondering what other health benefits you would get from the Sirtfood Diet, this is where we will discuss just that.

Weight Loss

The biggest factor behind the Sirtfood Diet's explosion in popularity is the fact that it promises rapid weight loss, whether you exercise or not. Given the fact that you undergo three(3) weeks of eating between 1,000 to 1,500 calories a day, of course, you will lose weight if you follow the diet to a T.

Keep in mind that an average person requires at least 2,000 calories a day, so you are eating anywhere between 50% to 75% of the required amount. Calorie deficit leads to weight loss. This weight loss is a mix of muscle and fat, sometimes water weight. As you continue to lose fat and muscle, your metabolism tends to slow down as well.

Therein lies the problem with some fasting diets. Over time, the weight loss plan would not be as effective as it claims to be. When your metabolism slows down, your body needs to burn fewer calories to function, so there would no longer be a calorie deficit. If you want to keep the weight loss momentum, you would need to cut down more calories. It's not hard to see how this is unsustainable.

Of course, as we've mentioned before, metabolism also plays a role in weight-loss. Sirtuin has already been proven to keep your metabolism up.

In other words, during the first two stages of the Sirtuin Diet, you would be having a calorie deficit while having your metabolism more or less at the same level, therefore accelerating the weight-loss process.

Positive Influence on Genetics

Here's a question that many of us probably have thought of at least once in our lives. Does fitness or thinness a genetic trait? Maybe you personally know someone with a large appetite who never gains weight no matter how much they eat or those who suddenly gain 7 pounds after eating a potato chip. If genetics have anything to do with this, does that mean losing weight is a matter of luck, a genetic dice roll, and no effort? Well, yes and no.

This is what has been referenced many times when someone pitches a speech on Sirtfood Diet. Although some people are truly blessed with such genetics, it is just a matter of when and how you activate your "skinny genes." Some people have them active since birth. Others may need a little help in activating them. They are in our DNA, after all. They are already in there. We just need to allow them to work.

We just need to let our cells know that it's not magic or science fiction. It's the truth. It's like a switch hidden behind a shelf. You just need to move the shelf away so you can access the switch and flip it.

Every single one of us has genes that can activate SIRTs or sirtuins. These are metabolism that controls how fast we burn through our fat and also regenerate cells. Think of them as if they are sensors that are triggered when our energy level is low. Most fasting-based diets rely on this mechanism. That's not to say that it doesn't have any drawback, however.

Perhaps the most popular form of fasting diet is intermittent fasting with all of its variants such as 16:8, 5:2, etc. In the 5:2 fasting regimen, you fast for two(2) days, usually on the weekends, and eat throughout the weekday as normal. It has been shown to improve your overall health and longevity, not to mention weight loss.

Fasting diets rely on the activation of the "skinny gene" in our body. When they are activated, the body goes into a power-saving mode by shutting down the fat-storage process and allows the body to burn up accumulated fat.

Fasting also has another beneficial effect on your cells. You see, whenever the cells in your body need to replicate, there is a very small chance that the DNA would be damaged in the process. This does not happen if your body repairs old or dying cells. For this reason, fasting is a way to lower your risk of developing neurodegenerative conditions such as Alzheimer's.

But there is one huge drawback, and that is the fact that you have to fast. Let's face it. It never feels good to be depriving your body of sustenance.

This problem is further compounded when you have to sit there without food while other people around you have a normal eating pattern.

You will be hungry while others are eating, not to mention that you would be put in a social spotlight when you have to explain to other people why you're not eating on certain days or times. Some people may even cast doubt or challenge your theory, saying that it's nothing but nonsense, which is a situation many people don't want to be in.

Moreover, although fasting has been proven to have many health benefits, there are some other downsides directly related to health as well. Fasting can lead to muscle loss. When the body needs to burn some extra energy and food isn't available, it could burn either body fat or muscle mass. It does not discriminate.

Other than that, there is the problem of malnutrition, which is to be expected when you don't eat enough food. Your body won't get enough essential nutrients. But this problem can be easily mitigated by taking supplements and eating nutrient-dense foods. Thankfully, Sirtfoods are full of nutrients.

Even so, fasting can slow or even stop the digestive system altogether, which may prevent the absorption of nutrients and supplements. In a strict fasting regimen, you may not get enough dietary fat, which supplements need to be dissolved.

Finally, fasting is certainly not for everyone. Children cannot fast because it will inhibit their growth. People who are ill need all the nutrients they can get so their bodies can fight off disease. Pregnant women need all the nutrients not for themselves but also for the infants. The elderly also need as many nutrients as they can get to sustain their aging bodies. These are the groups of people who should not fast.

There are many other psychological drawbacks to fasting, even though fasting is often associated with spiritual cleanliness. Fasting can put you slightly on edge or make you irritable. This is because your body is telling you that you need to forage for food, which is a very old instinct from the time when we actually need to hunt and forage for food. This activates certain physical processes that influence your mood and emotions, which may cause aggression.

Ever since its discovery in 1984, we now know that sirtuin activators boost activity in the mitochondria, which is the cell's powerhouse. This creates a boost in energy, which is an effect similar to that observed when you exercise or fast. The Sirtfood Diet is believed to kickstart a process that stops fat cells from duplicating, which is beneficial to dieters.

The best part is that sirtuin activators influence your genetics, debunking the belief that associates weight loss to genetic lottery. Genes are actually more flexible than you think. They can be changed. Of course, there isn't much you can do about the genes that determine the color of your eyes or your height, but you can influence the ones that control how much you gain or lose weight. You can enable or disable specific genes based on the external environment, which allows you to adapt. This is known as epigenetics, which is a fascinating subject in itself.

Keeping Appetite Under Control

During the first phase of the Sirtfood diet, you will feel very hungry because it is not used to having so few calories. However, your body will adjust and adapt to the new calorie restriction. It might take up to two weeks for some people, but you will eventually feel okay. Other than the calorie deficit, the

Sirtfoods you eat will be full of nutrients so your body would get all the nutrition it needs.

Preserve Muscle and Bone Mass

Sirtuins can also help boost muscle mass, especially for older people. This has been proven in an experiment conducted on much. They were fed foods rich in sirtuin, and it helped their development of blood vessels and muscle. This would lead to a boost in energy by up to 80%.

Metabolism and muscles go hand in hand. If you want your metabolism to stay up, you need to have your muscles in good condition as well. Otherwise, you may run into some health problems down the line. Therefore, you need a diet that at least preserves your muscle mass while still allowing you to lose weight, and the Sirtfood diet does just that.

Of course, maintaining your muscle mass also serves another purpose other than keeping you fit. It also keeps you looking nice and young as well.

Another important reason why muscle mass is so important has to do with how much energy your body burns as you are resting. Yes, you've read that right. Your body is always burning fuel. Think of it like your car with the engine running. Even if you're not driving, your car is always burning fuel so long as the engine is running. The only time when your body stops burning fuel is when you're no longer alive.

Your body also burns energy to digest food. Even when you're sleeping, your body burns energy, albeit at a much lower rate. It's just a matter of how much energy is burnt. Obviously, you would be burning many more calories when you're exercising compared to when you're just laying on the couch.

A large consumer of energy would be your muscles. Therefore, it follows that the more skeletal muscles you have, the more calories you burn, even when you're resting. Packing some extra muscles is like having a calorie safety net. You can eat a little bit more food and get away with it. Moreover, sirtuins help your heart health as it protects and strengthens your cardiac muscles and bones.

Blood Sugar Levels Under Control

Foods that are rich in sirtuins also help with improving blood sugar management by inhibiting the release of insulin. With sirtuins in your system, you can actually help prevent your blood sugar from getting too low. This is an important benefit you can get from Sirtfood Diet, especially if you are looking for a diet that can help stabilize your blood sugar level while also restricting your caloric intake.

You see, when you limit your caloric intake, your blood sugar level may drop. You will know this if you feel dizzy or weak if you ever skipped a meal or two. The lack of calories messes with your body's ability to manage blood sugar. Here, sirtuins can help regulate your blood sugar level so you can still function even when you've had only a little bit of food.

Better Sleep

Getting enough sleep is important as it reduces the chance of developing certain chronic diseases. An average adult needs to get somewhere between 7 to 8 hours of sleep a day. Of course, you can probably get away with a little bit of 6 hours of sleep, but getting enough sleep is critical for your health. It keeps the brain and digestive system healthy and also boosts your immune system.

How do sirtuins fit into this? Well, Sirtuin activators activate the SIR genes, which release SIRTs, or Silent Information Regulators. SIRTs help regulate the circadian rhythm. The circadian rhythm is your body's internal clock that tells you when it is time to sleep.

There was an interesting experiment in which the researcher locked himself up in a room with no way to tell the time, although he recorded when he went to bed and wake up. His sleeping pattern is more or less the same even though he didn't have a clock to tell him when it was time for bed. His internal clock regulated his sleeping patterns instead.

Sleep is probably one of the biggest things we underestimate, and it's not hard to see why. If you sleep for 8 hours a day for the rest of your life, you would be spending a third of your life sleeping. Some people just want to squeeze an extra hour or two, so they can do something else other than sleeping.

Sleep does a lot for the human body. It is crucial for many critical biological processes, such as those that help with regulating blood sugar levels that we've just discussed. That also contributes to losing weight as well. You know that your circadian rhythm is out of sync if you feel sleepy and in a state of brain fog all the time. Here, the Sirtfood Diet can help you restore balance and bring the rhythm back to normal.

Moreover, Sirtfoods contain certain ingredients that improve the quality of your sleep, such as almonds and chamomile tea. All of these have relaxing properties, so you can have a restful sleep and wake up the next day feeling refreshed and energetic.

Fight Off Free Radicals

Most Sirtfoods are full of antioxidants, and your body needs them to fight off chronic diseases such as cancer. Free radicals are the harmful by-products from being exposed to radiation or when your body breaks down food, and antioxidants are very useful in eliminating them. For this reason, eating Sirtfood can protect you from cancer, heart disease, and other common yet chronic diseases of the modern era.

Of course, a little bit of free radicals does not hurt, but they add up over time, and your body doesn't have the proper means to remove them on its own. Free radicals are a simple fact of life because even the sun has some degree of radiation, so you are exposed to it no matter where you go. Therefore, you need antioxidants to give your body the means to flush free radicals out, and many plant-based foodstuffs are full of them, especially Sirtfoods.

Reduced Stress and Anxieties

Stress and anxieties take up a lot of energy, but not in a way that would make you lose weight. Otherwise, emotional trauma would be the best way to lose weight. We're talking about mental energy here. Dealing with stress and anxieties can free up a lot of mental energy, allowing you to feel more at ease, among other benefits such as improving the quality of your sleep.

There are many ways to manage stress, such as hanging out with your friends, having regular meal times, etc. The Sirtfood Diet can also help you healthily cope with stress as Sirtfoods contain fatty fish, dark chocolate, eggs, pumpkin seeds, and Brazil nuts, all of which help reduce stress.

Anti-Aging Effects

As mentioned before, Sirtfood Diet helps to preserve muscle mass. This is a powerful way to protect against aging. As you grow older, your bones become weak and are more prone to breaking, and having more muscle mass help reinforce your bone and prevent bone fracture. Antioxidants, which help fight off free radicals, also help slow down the aging process.

Anti-aging is also linked to autophagy, which is a cell repair or replacement process. This process takes place inside a cell and it involves an enzyme called AMPK, which is essential for cellular energy homeostasis.

AMPK boosts energy by activating the fatty acid, glucose, and oxidation whenever the energy in the cell runs low. It is how the human body responds when there is a sharp spike in cellular energy demand. A similar effect is observed when you exert yourself when you exercise.

Part of this response is called lysosomal degradation autophagy. At this point, you might be wondering how sirtuins fit into all of this. You see, SIRT1 can also activate AMPK and vice versa, so SIRT1 is one way to trigger autophagy, which then regenerates the cells. This process can take place wherever on your body, from your muscles to your skin.

Triggering autophagy has a positive effect on your body and overall health, improving longevity since it repairs some of the damage caused by aging. Think of the process as taking your car to a mechanic. They will replace damaged or old parts and put in good ones, therefore allowing the car to run better for longer. Of course, the car will eventually be too old, and you will need to replace it.

The same goes for aging. There is no way to reverse aging or stop it altogether. There is no cure to aging, and autophagy isn't the fountain of youth either. The best you can do is slow down the aging process, allowing you to look younger than your age, although some effects associated with aging would still persist.

Fight Chronic Diseases

Although medicine is becoming more effective and complex, that does not necessarily mean that we are all getting healthier. Nowadays, around 70% of deaths are caused by chronic diseases.

It is shocking, true, but this has much to do with our lifestyles and what we put into our bodies. Most of such diseases can be avoided if we start eating healthy food. The rule of thumb is that the more processed the food, the less healthy it is. Thankfully, the damage caused by junk food can be reversed if you start eating healthy again, although it will take some time.

Many people's lifestyles and habits nowadays make it so easy to accumulate fat and other toxins, and the problem is further compounded when you bring in "convenient" foods that are full of sugar and saturated fat. This can easily lead to an increase in blood sugar and insulin levels. This is where the trouble begins as it causes pre-diabetes conditions that can lead to other chronic diseases.

The antidote to many of these ailments is already within us. It is the "skinny genes" that we've been discussing so far. Activating them could allow us to burn all that fat, expel all of those toxins, and allow our body to be strong and healthy once again.

Chapter 3: How to Get Started with the Sirtfood Diet When You're Over 50

The basic Sirtfood diet plan lasts for three(3) weeks and has 2 phases. After you have completed the 3-week trial, you can continue following the Sirtfood diet (or "sirtifying") for as long as you like by including as many Sirtfoods in your diet as possible.

As for the Sirtfood recipes themselves, there are plenty of resources online to help you get started. If you are worried about them using exotic and expensive ingredients, you don't have to worry much as most of the meals contain simple ingredients that are cheap and easy to find except for three(3) specific ingredients. Those are buckwheat, lovage, and matcha green tea powder. These can be scarce and expensive.

The majority of the diet is a green juice, which you will need to drink three(3) times a day. Again, the recipe can be found online.

With that out of the day, let's talk about the 2 phases of the Sirtfood diet that spans over three(3) weeks.

Phase One

This phase lasts for a week. The goal here is to kickstart your weight loss by putting tight restrictions on your caloric intake and introducing lots of green juice. According to the original author, you can lose as much as 7 pounds or 3.2kg in just seven(7) days.

For the first three(3) days, your caloric intake is limited to only 1,000 a day. That 1,000 calories are divided between the three(3) green juice and a Sirtfood meal. Sirtfood meals include shrimp stir-fry with buckwheat noodles, miso-glazed tofu, or the Sirtfood omelet.

From day 4 to 7, you can bump up your daily caloric intake to 1,500. You only need to drink green juice twice a day, and you can now have 2 Sirtfood meals. Again, the 1,500 calories are divided between the juice and meals.

It is here that some experts doubt the viability of the Sirtfood diet. Cutting your caloric intake down to 1,000 or even 1,500 is extreme for many people. They argue that weight-gain tends to bounce back after the first week because of slowed metabolism, among other things. This is where Phase Two of this diet comes in.

Phase Two

After the first week, you move on to phase 2 of the Sirtfood Diet. This is the maintenance phase, and you should continue to lose weight from here.

Unlike Phase One that places tight restrictions on your daily caloric intake, Phase Two does not do that.

Here, there is no specific calorie limit. You only need to drink the green juice once every day and can have 3 Sirtfood meals a day. All things being considered, this is where you start to ease your body back into your normal eating habits, except with Sirtfoods.

When to Stop

As mentioned, again and again, the Sirtfood Diet put tight calorie restriction for three(3) weeks. For a healthy adult, this should only cause a mild inconvenience. However, for those above the age of 50, there may be some more risks.

For this reason, it is best to keep a close eye on how you are feeling throughout the entirety of the 3-week program. You should only feel hungry, irritable, and light-headed at most. If any more serious symptoms show up, it is best to stop following this diet and consult a doctor.

Chapter 4: Foods You Can Eat on the Sirtfood Diet

Sirtfood Diet contains various foodstuffs that are known to increase the level of the sirtuin protein in your body. Such food is referred to as the

Sirtfoods, and among those are:

- Coffee
- Capers
- Blueberries
- Red Chicory
- Lovage
- Medjool dates
- Bird's eye chili
- Arugula
- Turmeric
- Walnuts
- Buckwheat
- Matcha green tea
- Extra virgin olive oil
- Dark chocolate (with 85% cocoa)
- Parsley
- Soy
- Onions
- Red wine
- Strawberries
- Kale

The above is considered as the top 20 Sirtfoods, so consider incorporating those into your diet as much as possible. There are countless online recipes out there to help you prepare sirtuin-rich food so you can get started.

You may be wondering what else you can eat other than the 20 foodstuffs we've mentioned above. Some nutritionists suggest that you should have some protein in addition to the Sirtfoods. Oily fish would be a good source of protein here. Just make sure to avoid fish that is rich in mercury. Other than that, consider incorporating dairy into your diet, but only in a moderate amount.

As you can see, the Sirtfood Diet doesn't have to be completely plant-based, although some people prefer going completely vegan with this diet.

Ideally, you don't want to focus on what food to cut out because most food groups have their own merit, other than processed and sugary foods, of course.

Other than that, you can incorporate some other foodstuffs into your Sirtfood Diet, although it is best to do it during the second phase when the calorie restriction is not so bad and that you get to eat 2 Sirtfood meals a day. After the second phase, you have even more freedom in choosing which food you want to eat. More on the phases later.

The foodstuffs mentioned above, such as cocoa nibs, dark chocolate, or walnuts, can be used as a Sirtfood snack to keep your energy and metabolism up throughout the day. Just make sure that you don't go over the calorie limit if you're within the first three(3) weeks of the program.

Chapter 5: How to Follow the Sirtfood Diet

As we've mentioned before, the Sirtfood Diet can be risky for the elderly as it puts a tight calorie restriction. This could lead to malnutrition and some other unseen health consequences. But what if you want to get some of that sirtuin effects, but you cannot follow the Sirtfood Diet? Are you doomed? No, not really.

The Sirtfood Diet demands calorie restriction for the first three(3) weeks. From there, you can have three(3) meals a day so long as those meals mainly comprise of Sirtfoods. For this reason, you can skip one or even both phases entirely and just focus on consuming Sirtfoods throughout the day.

The first three(3) weeks are intended to activate the sirtuins and other biological functions to help the body burn as much fat as possible. But as mentioned before, prolonged periods of fasting would slow down metabolism and nullify the effect of fasting. Think of the first three(3) weeks as the accelerated weight-loss program.

After the first week, metabolism should slow down a bit even with sirtuin in the system. So the move to a higher daily calorie allowance may slow down the weight-loss momentum a bit but still giving the body enough energy so that it would not slow down metabolism much more. After the second phase, or two(2) weeks, that would be time to move to a more stable and healthy diet and eating pattern.

By this point, the weight-loss momentum from fasting would be nullified, and metabolism may be slow. If you keep fasting for any longer, you may experience worse effects from fasting, and you wouldn't lose as much weight anyway. From there, you just need to eat Sirtfoods 3 times a day and drink the green juice once a day until your metabolism is good enough to allow you to repeat the 3-week program. You should give yourself at least a month's break from this before you attempt it again.

Therefore, if you cannot go through the 3-week program, you can just incorporate Sirtfoods into your daily meals. Of course, you won't experience the rapid weight loss that you would get if you commit yourself to the 3-week program. However, it would also be a lot easier to do since you won't be putting yourself through that ordeal.

Some may even say that it would be more sustainable if you just skip the 3-week program altogether. But it is highly recommended if you want to see results fast. You don't have to do it more than once if you don't want to. You are advised against doing it if your body is sending you a signal that something is wrong throughout the 3-week program.

Safety and Side Effects

As mentioned before, Sirtfood Diet may work for some people. The only way to know for sure is to give it a shot. You don't lose much anyway. But if you want to go into this, it is worth discussing the potential side effects you might experience. That way, you can decide whether you want to deal with them later on.

The biggest concern people have with Sirtfood Diet is the fact that it puts an extreme calorie restriction during the first week. Some nutrition experts also say that the diet itself is nutritionally incomplete for the first week. However, there is no real danger here since you don't have to stick with it for that one.

If you have diabetes, there may be some health concerns that arise from calorie restriction and drinking only juice for the first few days. There could be dangerous changes in blood sugar levels. If you have diabetes and want to try the Sirtfood diet, consider consulting your doctor or avoid it altogether.

Other than that, the only concern that you should have is hunger. This makes sense considering that you would only be eating 1,000 to 1,500 calories a day for the first three(3) weeks. Anyone would feel hungry. This is an expected side effect as you would only be drinking juice, which is low in fiber, a nutrient that keeps you feeling full.

You should experience some side effects only during the first week, which is Phase One of two in the Sirtfood Diet. You may experience fatigue, irritability, and lightheadedness, all of which are linked to the calorie restriction itself. Again, this is expected. Other health concerns are unlikely if you follow the diet for only three(3) weeks.

Chapter 6: Sirtfoods for Life

Although the basic Sirtfood Diet plan only lasts for two weeks, you can continue doing Phase Two for as long as you like. Alternatively, you can also repeat Phase One and move on to Phase Two as many times as you like for more weight loss, although you should not do it too often as 1,500 calories a day can take its toll on your body. You can do it once a month at most.

Some people are wondering whether you have to follow this for the rest of their lives. The answer is that they don't have to. Weight-loss, among other healthy habits, should be a fun process. If it is becoming a chore for you, then perhaps it is not for you or that you need a different approach.

The same applies to the Sirtfood Diet. If you don't feel good about it, then it is time to quit. But if you have been doing Phase Two for a while and things are starting to become bland, you can drop the diet and move on to other weight-loss diets or activities.

That said, you can incorporate Sirtfood Diet into your everyday meals, including the green juice. Of course, the effects would not be as prominent, but it is an easier alternative for those who can't or don't want to take up the Sirtfood diet in the first place.

For instance, you can also bring Sirtfood into other diets if you want to enjoy some benefits of the Sirtfood Diet. For instance, you can follow a vegan, gluten-free, paleo, or low-carb diet or even try out intermittent fasting while also consuming

Sirtfood. Bringing in Sirtfoods into the mix will only amplify the benefits of all of those diets.

This is how Sirtfood can provide various health benefits for a lifetime. In a way, Sirtfood is more than just a one-time diet. Going on a Sirtfood Diet requires you to change your lifestyle.

Is Sirtfoods the New Superfoods?

Let's get this out of the way first. Sirtfoods are good for you since they are rich in nutrients and healthy plant compounds. In addition, many health benefits are associated with Sirtfoods, based on various scientific studies.

For instance, having a moderate amount of dark chocolate that is rich in cocoa content can lower the risk of heart disease and fight inflammation. Green tea can also help lower the risk of stroke, diabetes and lower blood pressure. Tumeric also contains anti-inflammatory properties that can protect against diseases associated with chronic inflammation, among other health benefits.

Overall, most of the Sirtfoods provide health benefits for humans. That said, we do not have enough evidence on the health benefits from increasing the sirtuin levels in humans, although experiments conducted on animals showed positive results. For instance, increasing sirtuin levels in mice, worms, and yeast lead to better longevity.

Additionally, sirtuins have a special effect on the body when you are fasting or undergoing calorie restriction. The protein tells the body to burn up more fat for energy while also improving insulin sensitivity. This study has been conducted on mice, and it led to weight loss.

Other evidence also suggests that sirtuins may help fight inflammation, slow tumor development, and slow the development of Alzheimer's and heart disease.

Other scientific research has been conducted on mice and human cell lines, and those have also shown positive results. To this day, there have been no scientific studies conducted on humans directly.

As such, we still do not have a definitive answer as to whether increasing the sirtuin levels in the human body can lead longer lifespan, although various experiments conducted on cells showed promising results. But maybe we don't have to wait for too long for an answer as there is already research underway to create compounds that are effective in increasing sirtuins levels in the human body. If this is successful, human studies can be conducted.

In short, are Sirtfoods and the diet regimen worth it? The foods themselves are definitely healthy. The research so far all suggest that the Sirtfood diet is effective. The scientists just need a bit more time to give us a definitive answer when they can conduct human studies.

Is it Healthy and Sustainable?

The biggest problem with some fad diet is the fact that they promise quick weight-loss that is usually very unhealthy and unsustainable. If you follow such a diet, you will end up gaining more weight after you cannot keep up with the diet or transition to a normal diet again.

Generally, the problem with such diet is that they restrict the caloric intake too much, therefore causing the body's metabolism to slow down, burning less body fat while making you feel terrible at the same time. The basic equation to losing weight is to burn more calorie than you consume, which force the body to burn its fat store for energy. So to lose weight quickly, you consume very little amount of calories, right? No.

Losing weight is more nuanced than that. You see, when you do not get your usual amount of calories, your body thinks that your life is in danger. It thinks that food may be scarce going forward, and so it goes into a "power saving mode" by drastically lowering the metabolism rate, therefore causing your body to use much less energy and burn up much less body fat.

This power-saving mode persists until you start eating normally again. The problem is that when you do, your body attempts to replenish its fat store by keeping the metabolism rate low while still absorbing a lot of calories, leading to weight gain again. More often than not, you gain more weight than you lose in a short period that you spent following the unsustainable diet plan.

As Sirtfood Diet severely restricts your daily caloric intake to only 1,500 calories, which some experts say is extreme to many people, this begs the question of whether the diet is actually healthy and sustainable.

First, let's discuss the foods that are considered to be Sirtfoods. Most of them are healthy options and are linked to various health benefits since they have anti-inflammatory and antioxidant properties. That said, eating some healthy food does not provide your body with all its nutritional needs.

So we have come to this assessment. The Sirtfood Diet is very restrictive calorie-wise and does not provide unique or clear health benefits that other diet regimens offer. Experts do not recommend having only 1,000 calories a day unless under the supervision of a physician. 1,500 calories a day is still quite restrictive for many people.

A signature food in the Sirtfood Diet is the green juice, which you need to drink up to 3 times a day until you start to wane off the juice after the first week. Of course, the juice is a good source of minerals and vitamins, but it also contains sugar and no healthy fiber that veggies and whole fruits contain. As it contains sugar, drinking green juice throughout the day can be bad for your teeth and blood sugar level as well.

Many people are doubtful about the Sirtfood Diet primarily because of the restrictions during the first week. Your choices for Sirtfoods aren't that generous either, so you may have to take supplements to make up for the deficiency in proteins, vitamins, and minerals. In addition, you may have to purchase a juicer to make the green juice and some expensive ingredients to make your Sirtfoods.

With all this in mind, it is one of the diets that is difficult for many people to follow for three(3) whole weeks. In a perfect world, we would only have a universal diet plan that guarantees weight-loss. However, not all diets work for everyone. Our bodies are built differently, and they react differently to even the same diet. So, there really is no one-size-fits-all diet here.

The same applies to the Sirtfood diet. It may not be anyone's first choice for diet, but if every other diet plan you've tried does not work for you, then it's worth giving Sirtfood Diet a shot. It could work for you, or maybe it couldn't. It depends on how your body handles it.

Summary

In short, the Sirtfood Diet is low in calories, and the first phase is definitely not nutritionally balanced. You will feel hungry and tired, but you shouldn't experience anything worse than that. Consult a doctor or a physician immediately if any more serious symptoms arise.

Many people are skeptical because the Sirtfood Diet does not allow for a healthy eating pattern for the first phase, although it contains a lot of healthy food. The science is still uncertain about whether this is a viable way to lose weight, not to mention that the diet itself may contain ingredients that are expensive or hard to acquire. It is definitely not a diet for everyone, although it's worth a shot if all other alternatives prove ineffective for you.

Breakfast Recipes

Cherry and Banana Smoothie

Prep Time: 5 minutes; Cooking Time: 0 minutes; Yields: 1 glass;

Ingredients:

½ cup almond milk, unsweetened

1 large banana, frozen

1 cup frozen cherries

1 teaspoon of cocoa powder

1 tablespoon peanut butter

Directions:

Place all the ingredients into the jar of a high-speed food processor or blender in the order stated in the ingredients list and then cover it with the lid.

Pulse for 1 minute until smooth and then serve.

Nutritional Information per Serving:

Calories: 292.9 Cal; Fat: 4.4 g; Protein: 14.7 g; Carbs: 52.5 g; Fiber: 3.9 g;

Banana and Green Smoothie

Prep Time: 5 minutes; Cooking Time: 0 minutes; Yields: 1 glass;

Ingredients:

1 cup of coconut water

¾ cup almond milk, unsweetened

1 cup spinach leaves, fresh

3 cups sliced bananas, frozen

¼ teaspoon vanilla extract, unsweetened

½ tablespoon coconut sugar

Directions:

Place all the ingredients into the jar of a high-speed food processor or blender in the order stated in the ingredients list and then cover it with the lid.

Pulse for 1 minute until smooth and then serve.

Nutritional Information per Serving:

Calories: 177.1 Cal; Fat: 3.8 g; Protein: 13.4 g; Carbs: 26 g; Fiber: 3.4 g;

Breakfast Burrito

Prep Time: 5 minutes; Cooking Time: 10 minutes; Yields: 4 burritos;

Ingredients:

12 ounces extra-firm tofu, pressed, drained

½ cup diced white onion

1 cup baby spinach, fresh

½ cup diced red bell pepper

½ teaspoon of sea salt

2 teaspoons ground turmeric

2 teaspoons nutritional yeast

1 teaspoon Worcestershire sauce

3 tablespoons vegetable broth

4 whole-grain tortillas

Directions:

Place the drained tofu in a medium bowl and then crumble it, set aside until required.

Pour the broth into a medium frying pan, place it over medium heat and when hot, add onion and bell pepper.

Stir until mixed and then cook for 3 minutes or until sauté.

Add crumbled tofu along with yeast, turmeric, and Worcestershire sauce, stir until mixed, and then continue cooking for 3 minutes.

Stir in spinach, cover the pan with its lid, and then leave the spinach leaves wilt for 3 minutes.

Divide the tofu mixture evenly among the tortillas, fold each tortilla and then serve.

Nutritional Information per Serving:

Calories: 254.8 Cal; Fat: 11.1 g; Protein: 23.1 g; Carbs: 33.9 g; Fiber: 10 g;

Chocolate Waffles

Prep Time: 5 minutes; Cooking Time: 10 minutes; Yields: 2 waffles;

Ingredients:

1 cup whole-wheat flour

1 ½ cup cooked black beans

2 bananas, peeled

2 teaspoons baking powder

½ cup of cocoa powder

7 tablespoons maple syrup

½ cup chocolate chips

¾ cup almond milk, unsweetened

Directions:

Place the black beans in a blender, add banana, maple syrup, cocoa powder, and milk and then pulse until smooth.

Add baking powder and flour into the blender and then pulse until just combined.

Spoon the batter into a bowl and then fold in chocolate chips until just mixed.

Switch on the waffle maker and then let it preheat.

Pour the batter into the waffle maker, shut with its lid, and then cook for 3 to 5 minutes until firm.

Transfer the cooked waffle to a plate and then repeat with the remaining batter.

Serve straight away with berries.

Nutritional Information per Serving:

Calories: 127 Cal; Fat: 6 g; Protein: 2 g; Carbs: 18 g; Fiber: 6 g;

Pumpkin and Berries Quinoa

Prep Time: 4 hours and 5 minutes; Cooking Time: 0 minutes; Yields: 1 bowl;

Ingredients:

½ cup chopped strawberries

1 cup oats, old-fashioned

3 tablespoons pumpkin seeds

1 cup almond milk, unsweetened

Directions:

Place oats in a bowl, add berries and pumpkin seeds and then pour in the milk.

Cover the bowl with its lid and then refrigerate for a minimum of 4 hours.

Stir the oats and then serve.

Nutritional Information per Serving:

Calories: 142 Cal; Fat: 2 g; Protein: 4 g; Carbs: 27 g; Fiber: 3 g;

Chocolate, Peanut Butter and Chickpea Pancakes

Prep Time: 5 minutes; Cooking Time: 15 minutes; Yields: 30 pancakes, 4 pancakes per serving;

Ingredients:

2 cups cooked chickpeas

2 tablespoons flax meal

½ cup dark chocolate chips

1 teaspoon baking soda

1 teaspoon ground cinnamon

1 teaspoon vanilla extract, unsweetened

1/3 cup peanut butter

1 tablespoon olive oil

4 tablespoons applesauce

½ cup almond milk, unsweetened

4 ½ tablespoons water, warm

.

Directions:

Take a small bowl, place flax meal in it, stir in water until mixed, and then set aside for 5 minutes until mixture resembles gel. .

Place chickpeas in a food processor, add applesauce and then pulse until smooth.

Add remaining ingredients, reserving chocolate chips, and then pulse until smooth batter comes together.

Tip the mixture into a large bowl, stir in chocolate chips and then stir until well incorporated.

Take a large skillet pan, place it over medium heat, add oil and when hot, scoop 1/8 cup of the batter per pancake in it.

Shape the batter into a pancake and then cook for 2 to 3 minutes per side until cooked.

Transfer the pancake to a plate and then serve.

Nutritional Information per Serving:

Calories: 292 Cal; Fat: 14.1 g; Protein: 8.1 g; Carbs: 34.1 g; Fiber: 3 g;

Kale Wrapped Eggs

Prep Time: 8-10 min.

Cooking Time: 5 min.

Number of Servings: 4

Ingredients:

Three tablespoons heavy cream

Four hardboiled eggs

¼ teaspoon pepper

Four kale leaves

Four prosciutto slices

¼ teaspoon salt

1 ½ cups water

Directions:

1. Peel the eggs and wrap each with the kale. Wrap them in the prosciutto slices and sprinkle with ground black pepper and salt.

2. Arrange Instant Pot over a dry platform in your kitchen. Open its top lid and switch it on.

3. In the pot, pour water. Arrange a trivet or steamer basket inside that came with Instant Pot. Now place/arrange the eggs over the trivet/basket.
4. Close the lid to create a locked chamber; make sure that safety valve is in locking position.
5. Find and press "MANUAL" cooking function; timer to 5 minutes with default "HIGH" pressure mode.
6. Allow the pressure to build to cook the ingredients.
7. After cooking time is over press "CANCEL" setting. Find and press "QPR" cooking function. This setting is for quick release of inside pressure.
8. Slowly open the lid, take out the cooked recipe in serving plates or serving bowls, and enjoy the keto recipe.

Nutritional Information per Serving:

Calories – 247; Fat – 20g; Carbs – 7g; Fiber – 3g; Protein – 19g

Artichoke Dip

Prep Time: 5 minutes; Cooking Time: 5 minutes; Servings: 20;

Ingredients:

Frozen spinach – 10-ounce

Artichoke hearts, chopped – 14 ounce

Cloves of garlic, peeled – 3

Onion powder – 1 teaspoon

Mayonnaise, full-fat – ½ cup

Parmesan cheese, grated and full-fat – 12 ounces

Cream cheese, full-fat – 8 ounces

Sour cream, full-fat – ½ cup

Swiss cheese, grated, full-fat – 12 ounces

Chicken broth, organic – ½ cup

Directions:

Switch on an instant pot, place all the ingredients except for Swiss cheese and parmesan cheese and stir until just mixed.

Shut instant pot with its lid, sealed completely, press manual button and cook eggs for 4 minutes at high pressure.

When done, let the pressure release naturally for 5 minutes, then do quick pressure release and open the instant pot.

Add Swiss and parmesan cheese into the instant pot and stir well until cheeses melt and is well combined.

Serve immediately.

Nutritional Info:

Calories: 230.7; Fat: 18.7 g; Protein: 12.6 g; Net Carbs: 2.6 g; Fiber: 0.7 g;

Zucchini Noodles

Prep Time: 5 minutes; Cooking Time: 6 minutes; Servings: 2;

Ingredients:

Medium zucchini, spiralized into noodles – 2

Butter, unsalted – 2 tablespoons

Minced garlic – 1 ½ tablespoon

Parmesan cheese, grated – 3/4 cup

Sea salt – ½ teaspoon

Ground black pepper – ¼ teaspoon

Red chili flakes – ¼ teaspoon

Directions:

Switch on the instant pot, add butter, press the 'sauté/simmer' button, wait until the butter melts, and add garlic and cook for 1 minute or until fragrant.

Add zucchini noodles, toss until coated, cook for 5 minutes or until tender and season with salt and black pepper.

Press the 'keep warm' button, then transfer to noodles to a dish, top with cheese and sprinkle with red chili flakes.

Serve straight away.

Nutritional Info:

Calories: 298; Fat: 26.1 g; Protein: 5 g; Net Carbs: 2.3 g; Fiber: 0.1 g;

Grapes and Green Tea Smoothie

Prep Time: 5 minutes; Cooking Time: 0 minutes; Yields: 2 glasses;

Ingredients:

½ cup green tea

½ cup of green grapes

1 banana, peeled

1-inch piece of ginger

½ cup of ice cubes

2 cups baby spinach

½ of a medium apple, peeled, diced

Directions:

Place all the ingredients into the jar of a high-speed food processor or blender in the order stated in the ingredients list and then cover it with the lid.

Pulse for 1 minute until smooth, and then serve.

Nutritional Information per Serving:

Calories: 150 Cal; Fat: 2.5 g; Protein: 1 g; Carbs: 36.5 g; Fiber: 9 g;

Mango and Kale Smoothie

Prep Time: 5 minutes; Cooking Time: 0 minutes; Yields: 2 glasses;

Ingredients:

2 cups oats milk, unsweetened

2 bananas, peeled

½ cup kale leaves

2 teaspoons coconut sugar

1 cup mango pieces

1 teaspoon vanilla extract, unsweetened

Directions:

Place all the ingredients into the jar of a high-speed food processor or blender in the order stated in the ingredients list and then cover it with the lid.

Pulse for 1 minute until smooth, and then serve.

Nutritional Information per Serving:

Calories: 281 Cal; Fat: 3 g; Protein: 6 g; Carbs: 63 g; Fiber: 16 g;

Pomegranate Smoothie

Prep Time: 5 minutes; Cooking Time: 0 minutes; Yields: 2 glasses;

Ingredients:

2 cups almond milk, unsweetened

2 medium apples, cored, sliced

2 bananas, peeled

2 cups frozen raspberries

1 cup pomegranate seeds

4 teaspoons agave syrup

Directions:

Place all the ingredients into the jar of a high-speed food processor or blender in the order stated in the ingredients list and then cover it with the lid.

Pulse for 1 minute until smooth, and then serve.

Nutritional Information per Serving:

Calories: 141.5 Cal; Fat: 1.1 g; Protein: 4.1 g; Carbs: 30.8 g; Fiber: 2.4 g;

Zucchini and Blueberry Smoothie

Prep Time: 5 minutes; Cooking Time: 0 minutes; Yields: 2 glasses;

Ingredients:

1 cup coconut milk, unsweetened

1 large celery stem

2 bananas, peeled

½ cup spinach leaves, fresh

1 cup frozen blueberries

2/3 cup sliced zucchini

1 tablespoon hemp seeds

½ teaspoon maca powder

¼ teaspoon ground cinnamon

Directions:

Place all the ingredients into the jar of a high-speed food processor or blender in the order stated in the ingredients list and then cover it with the lid.

Pulse for 1 minute until smooth, and then serve.

Nutritional Information per Serving:

Calories: 218 Cal; Fat: 10.1 g; Protein: 6.3 g; Carbs: 31.8 g; Fiber: 4.7 g;

Hot Pink Beet Smoothie

Prep Time: 5 minutes; Cooking Time: 0 minutes; Yields: 2 glasses;

Ingredients:

2 cups almond milk, unsweetened

2 clementine, peeled

1 cup raspberries

1 banana, peeled

1 medium beet, peeled, chopped

2 tablespoons chia seeds

1/8 teaspoon sea salt

½ teaspoon vanilla extract, unsweetened

4 tablespoons almond butter

Directions:

Place all the ingredients into the jar of a high-speed food processor or blender in the order stated in the ingredients list and then cover it with the lid.

Pulse for 1 minute until smooth, and then serve.

Nutritional Information per Serving:

Calories: 260.8 Cal; Fat: 1.3 g; Protein: 13 g; Carbs: 56 g; Fiber: 9.3 g;

Vegetable Pancakes

Prep Time: 10 minutes; Cooking Time: 20 minutes; Yields: 10 Pancakes;

Ingredients:

1/3 cup cooked and mashed sweet potato

2 cups grated carrots

1 cup chopped coriander

1 cup cooked spinach

3.5 ounces chickpea flour

½ teaspoon baking powder

1 ½ teaspoon salt

1 teaspoon ground turmeric

2 tablespoons olive oil

¾ cup of water

Directions:

Take a large bowl, place chickpea flour in it, add turmeric powder, baking powder, and salt, and then stir until combined. Whisk in the water until combined, stir in sweet potatoes until well mixed and then add carrots, spinach, and coriander until well combined.

Take a large skillet pan, place it over medium-high heat, add 1 tablespoon oil and then let it heat.

Scoop the pancake mixture in portions into the pan, shape each portion like a pancake and then cook for 3 to 5 minutes per side until pancakes turn golden brown and thoroughly cooked.

When done, transfer the pancakes to a plate, add more oil into the pan and then cook more pancakes in the same manner.

Serve straight away.

Nutritional Information per Serving:

Calories: 74 Cal; Fat: 0.3 g; Protein: 3 g; Carbs: 16 g; Fiber: 2.7 g;

Lunch Recipes

Lentil and Quinoa Salad

Prep Time: 5 minutes; Cooking Time: 15 minutes; Yields: 6 bowls;

Ingredients:

2 medium green apples, cored, chopped

3 cups cooked quinoa

½ of a medium red onion, peeled, diced

3 cups cooked green lentils

1 large carrot, shredded

1 ½ teaspoon salt

1 teaspoon ground black pepper

2 tablespoons olive oil

¼ cup balsamic vinegar

Directions:

Take a large bowl, place all the ingredients in it and then stir until combined.

Let the salad chill in the refrigerator for 1 hour, divide it evenly among six bowls and then serve.

Nutritional Information per Serving:

Calories: 199 Cal; Fat: 10.7 g; Protein: 8 g; Carbs: 34.8 g; Fiber: 5.9 g;

Ginger Brown Rice

Prep Time: 5 minutes; Cooking Time: 40 minutes; Yields: 3 bowls;

Ingredients:

1 cup brown rice, rinsed

1-inch grated ginger

½ of serrano pepper, chopped

1 green onion, chopped

2 cups of water

Directions:

Take a medium pot, place it over medium-high heat, and then pour in water.

Add rice, green onion, serrano pepper, and ginger, bring to a boil, switch heat to medium and then simmer for 30 minutes.

Divide rice among three bowls and then serve.

Nutritional Information per Serving:

Calories: 125 Cal; Fat: 1 g; Protein: 3 g; Carbs: 26 g; Fiber: 0 g;

Chickpea Salad

Prep Time: 5 minutes; Cooking Time: 0 minutes; Yields: 2 servings;

Ingredients:

1 cup cooked chickpeas

16 leaves of butter lettuce

1 cup chopped zucchini

½ spring onion, chopped

1 cup chopped celery

1 cup grated carrot

1 tablespoon chopped cilantro

½ teaspoon salt

½ tablespoon lemon juice

Directions:

Take a large bowl, place all the ingredients in it, toss until mixed, and let it sit for 15 minutes.

Divide the lettuce leaves between two portions, top with the salad evenly and then serve.

Nutritional Information per Serving:

Calories: 166.6 Cal; Fat: 7.7 g; Protein: 4.4 g; Carbs: 20.8 g; Fiber: 4.3 g;

Kale Tacos

Prep Time: 10 minutes; Cooking Time: 10 minutes; Yields: 8 tacos;

Ingredients:

1 cup cooked black beans

1 cup chopped kale

½ of a medium avocado, sliced

1 cup chopped white onion

1 cup chopped tomatoes

2 tablespoons chopped cilantro

½ teaspoon minced garlic

2/3 teaspoon salt

½ of a lemon

1 tablespoon water

8 small tacos

Directions:

Place beans in a medium bowl, add salt, cumin powder, and then mash by using a fork until beans have broken.

Take a medium skillet pan, place it over medium heat, add water, add kale and garlic, then cook for 4 minutes or until softened, set aside until required.

Heat the tacos until thoroughly warmed, fold each taco in half, spread 1 tablespoon of bean mixture on one-half side of taco, and then top

with tomatoes, onion, avocado, kale, and cilantro.

Drizzle with lemon juice, fold, and then serve.

Nutritional Information per Serving:

Calories: 109.9 Cal; Fat: 2.9 g; Protein: 4.9 g; Carbs: 17 g; Fiber: 5 g;

Chickpea and Avocado Salad

Prep Time: 5 minutes; Cooking Time: 0 minutes; Yields: 4 servings;

Ingredients:

1 ½ cup cooked chickpeas

1 medium avocado

¼ teaspoon salt

¼ teaspoon ground black pepper

¼ cup chopped cilantro

2 tablespoons chopped green onion

3 tablespoons lime juice

Directions:

Place chickpeas in a medium bowl and then mash with a fork.

Add avocado into the chickpeas, mash with a fork, add green onion and cilantro, drizzle with lime juice, and season with salt and black pepper.

Serve the chickpea salad on bread as a sandwich.

Nutritional Information per Serving:

Calories: 234 Cal; Fat: 8 g; Protein: 10 g; Carbs: 33 g; Fiber: 11 g;

Spinach and Orange Salad

Prep Time: 5 minutes; Cooking Time: 0 minutes; Yields: 6 serving;

Ingredients:

10 ounces fresh spinach

1 teaspoon Brazil nuts

10 strawberries, sliced

1 teaspoon sunflower seeds

10 ounces canned clementine oranges

¼ cup raspberry vinaigrette

Directions:

Take a medium bowl, place all the ingredients in it and then toss until coated.

Serve straight away.

Nutritional Information per Serving:

Calories: 109 Cal; Fat: 2 g; Protein: 3 g; Carbs: 18 g; Fiber: 4 g;

Roasted Tomatoes

Prep Time: 5 minutes; Cooking Time: 25 minutes; Yields: 3 servings;

Ingredients:

3 ½ cups halved cherry tomatoes

3 teaspoons minced garlic

½ teaspoon salt

1 tablespoon minced basil

¼ teaspoon red chili flakes

½ teaspoon balsamic vinegar

1 tablespoon olive oil

1 tablespoon minced parsley

Directions:

Switch on the oven, then set it to 375 degrees F and let it preheat.

Take a large bowl, place all the ingredients in it and then toss until mixed.

Take a baking sheet, line it with a parchment sheet, spread tomato mixture, and then bake for 25 minutes until roasted.

Serve straight away.

Nutritional Information per Serving:

Calories: 115.6 Cal; Fat: 9.6 g; Protein: 1.6 g; Carbs: 8 g; Fiber: 1.6 g;

Asparagus Soup

Prep Time: 5 minutes; Cooking Time: 28 minutes; Yields: 6 bowls;

Ingredients:

4 pounds potatoes, peeled, chopped

1 bunch of asparagus

15 ounces cooked cannellini beans

1 small white onion, peeled, diced

3 teaspoons minced garlic

1 teaspoon grated ginger

½ teaspoon salt

¼ teaspoon ground black pepper

1 lemon, juiced

1 tablespoon olive oil

8 cups vegetable broth

Directions:

Place oil in a large pot, place it over medium heat and let it heat until hot.

Add onion into the pot, stir in garlic and ginger and then cook for 5 minutes until onion turns tender.

Add potatoes, asparagus, and beans, pour in the broth, stir until mixed, and then bring the mixture to a boil.

Cook the potatoes for 20 minutes until tender, remove the pot from heat and then puree half of the soup until smooth.

Add salt, black pepper, and lemon juice, stir until mixed, ladle soup into bowls and then serve.

Nutritional Information per Serving:

Calories: 123.3 Cal; Fat: 4.4 g; Protein: 4.7 g; Carbs: 16.3 g; Fiber: 4.1 g;

Roasted Brussel Sprouts

Prep Time: 5 minutes; Cooking Time: 30 minutes; Yields: 4 servings;

Ingredients:

3 cups Brussel sprouts

½ cup dried cranberries

1 ½ teaspoon salt

1 teaspoon ground black pepper

2 tablespoons olive oil

Directions:

Switch on the oven, then set it to 375 degrees F and let it preheat.

Meanwhile, cut each Brussel sprout in half and then place them in a large bowl.

Add salt and black pepper, drizzle with oil, toss until coated, and then spread on a baking sheet.

Add cranberries to it, and then roast the Brussel sprouts for 30 minutes until cooked.

Serve straight away.

Nutritional Information per Serving:

Calories: 135 Cal; Fat: 9.8 g; Protein: 3.9 g; Carbs: 11 g; Fiber: 4 g;

Green Bean Casserole

Prep Time: 10 minutes; Cooking Time: 30 minutes; Yields: 6 servings;

Ingredients:

1 ½ cups diced cremini mushrooms

1 cup of frozen green beans

6-ounce fried onions

2 teaspoons minced garlic

½ cup diced white onion

3 ½ tablespoons white whole-wheat flour

½ teaspoon dried oregano

3 ½ tablespoons olive oil

2 cups vegetable broth

Directions:

Switch on the oven, then set it to 400 degrees F and let it preheat.

Take a medium saucepan, place it over medium heat, add oil, and let it heat.

Add mushrooms and onion, stir in garlic and then cook for 4 minutes or until softened.

Stir in flour until smooth, cook for 2 minutes until golden and then stir in vegetable broth.

Simmer the mixture for 5 minutes, stir in black pepper and oregano and continue cooking for 10 to 15 minutes until gravy reach to desire thickness, stirring gently.

Stir in green beans and then spoon the mixture into a skillet pan.

Top the bean mixture with fried onions and then bake for 15 minutes until done.

Serve straight away.

Nutritional Information per Serving:

Calories: 191 Cal; Fat: 10 g; Protein: 4.1 g; Carbs: 22 g; Fiber: 3.3 g;

Kale Chips

Prep Time: 5 minutes; Cooking Time: 12 minutes; Servings: 4;

Ingredients:

Large bunch of organic kale – 1

Seasoned salt – 1 tablespoon

Olive oil – 2 tablespoons

Directions:

Set oven to 350 degrees F and preheat.

Meanwhile, separate kale leaves from its stem, rinse the leaves under running water, then drain completely by using a vegetable spinner.

Wipe kale leaves with paper towels to remove excess water, then transfer them into a large plastic bag and add oil.

Seal the plastic bag, turn it upside down until kale is coated with oil and then spread kale leaves on a large baking sheet.

Place the baking sheet into the oven and bake for 12 minutes or until its edges are nicely golden brown.

Remove baking sheet from the oven, season kale with salt and serve. .

Nutritional Info:

Calories: 163; Fat: 10 g; Protein: 2 g; Net Carbs: 14 g; Fiber: 2 g;

Guacamole

Prep Time: 10 minutes; Cooking Time: 0 minutes; Servings: 4;

Ingredients:

Organic avocados, pitted – 2

Medium organic red onion, peeled and sliced – 1/3

Medium organic jalapeño, deseeded and diced – 1

Salt – ½ teaspoon

Ground pepper – ½ teaspoon

Tomato salsa, organic – 2 tablespoons

Lime juice, organic – 1 tablespoon

Bunch of organic cilantro – ½

Directions:

Cut each avocado into half, remove its pit and slice its flesh horizontally and vertically.

Scoop out the flesh of the avocado, place it in a bowl and add onion, jalapeno, and lime juice then stir until well mixed.

Season with salt and black pepper, add salsa and stir with a fork until avocado is mash to desired consistency.

Fold in cilantro and serve.

Nutritional Info:

Calories: 16.5; Fat: 1.4 g; Protein: 0.23 g; Net Carbs: 0.5 g; Fiber: 0.6 g;

Brussels Sprout Skewers

Prep Time: 10 minutes; Cooking Time: 20 minutes; Yields: 4;

Ingredients:

½ of a medium red onion, peeled, sliced into 1-inch squares

1 pound Brussels sprouts, halved

¼ teaspoon of sea salt

1 tablespoon maple syrup

3 tablespoons balsamic vinegar

1 tablespoon Dijon mustard

3 tablespoons olive oil

Directions:

Take a large pot half full with water, place it over medium-high heat and then bring it to a boil.

Add Brussel sprouts, cook for 1 minute until tender, remove them from the pot, rinse well until cold water and then pat dry with paper towels.

Transfer Brussel sprouts in a large bowl, add onion and remaining ingredients, and then toss until coated.

Take a griddle pan, place it over medium-high heat, grease it with oil and then let it heat until hot.

Thread Brussel sprouts and onions on skewers, four sprouts per skewer, and then brush with remaining marinade.

Arrange the prepared skewers onto the grill pan and then cook for 7 to 10 minutes per side until vegetables turn nicely brown.

Serve straight away.

Nutritional Information per Serving:

Calories: 159.3 Cal; Fat: 10.5 g; Protein: 3.9 g; Carbs: 13.2 g; Fiber: 4.5 g;

Quinoa Tacos

Prep Time: 10 minutes; Cooking Time: 35 minutes; Yields: 10 tacos;

Ingredients:

½ of medium red bell pepper, cored, sliced

1 cup quinoa

½ of medium orange bell pepper, cored, sliced

2 green onions

4 cups mixed greens

1 teaspoon onion powder

1 teaspoon garlic powder

½ teaspoon salt, divided

1 tablespoon cumin powder

1 teaspoon dried oregano

1 tablespoon paprika

3 tablespoons coconut oil

2 cups vegetable broth

2 tablespoons lime juice

12 tablespoons cashew cream

12 tablespoons salsa

12 corn tortillas

Directions:

Cook the quinoa, and for this, take a medium saucepan, place it over medium heat and let it heat until hot.

Add quinoa, cook for 3 to 4 minutes until toasted, transfer quinoa to a strainer, and then rinse it well.

Return quinoa into the saucepan, pour in the vegetable broth, stir in ¼ teaspoon salt and then bring quinoa to boil.

Switch heat to the low level, cover the pan with its lid and then simmer quinoa for 15 to 20 minutes until the quinoa has absorbed all the liquid.

Meanwhile, take a medium bowl, place red bell pepper slices in it, drizzle with 1 tablespoon of lime juice, toss until coated, and then set aside until required.

When done, remove the saucepan from heat, let the quinoa rest for 5 minutes, uncover the pan and then fluff with a fork.

Take a large skillet pan, place it over medium heat, add oil and let it heat until melted.

Add quinoa, stir until combined, stir in remaining salt, onion powder, garlic powder, cumin, and paprika and then cook for 5 minutes until bottom begins to turn crisp, don't stir.

Remove pan from heat, add green onions and remaining lime juice, and stir until mixed.

Assemble the tacos and for this, warm the tortillas until hot and slightly blacken and then fill evenly with mixed greens.

Stuff the tortillas with quinoa mixture, red bell peppers, salsa, and cashew cream, and then serve.

Nutritional Information per Serving:

Calories: 150.5 Cal; Fat: 5.2 g; Protein: 4 g; Carbs: 23.3 g; Fiber: 3.5 g;

Ginger Veggie Stir-Fry

Prep Time: 5 minutes; Cooking Time: 10 minutes; Yields: 6;

Ingredients:

1 small head of broccoli, cut into florets

¾ cup julienned carrots

¼ cup chopped white onion

½ cup halved green beans

½ cup snow peas

1 teaspoon minced garlic

2 teaspoons grated ginger, divided

½ tablespoon salt

1 tablespoon cornstarch

2 tablespoons soy sauce

¼ cup olive oil, divided

2 ½ tablespoons water

Directions:

Take a large bowl, place 1 teaspoon grated ginger in it, add 2 tablespoons of olive oil, garlic, and cornstarch and then whisk well until cornstarch has dissolved.

Add green beans, carrots, snow peas, and broccoli florets, and then toss until coated.

Take a large skillet pan, place it over medium heat, add remaining oil and when hot, add vegetables and then cook for 2 minutes, tossing frequently.

Add soy sauce and water into the pan along with onion and remaining ginger, season with salt, and then continue cooking for 3 to 4 minutes until vegetables turn tender-crisp.

Serve straight away.

Nutritional Information per Serving:

Calories: 118.6 Cal; Fat: 9.3 g; Protein: 2.2 g; Carbs: 8 g; Fiber: 2.2 g;

Dinner Recipes

Eggplant and Potatoes in Tomato Sauce

Prep Time: 5 minutes; Cooking Time: 15 minutes; Yields: 4;

Ingredients:

3 large potatoes, boiled, cut into cubes

14 ounces crushed tomatoes

1 medium eggplant, destemmed, cut into cubes

2 tablespoons minced garlic

1 teaspoon salt

1 tablespoon curry powder

1 tablespoon soy sauce

3 tablespoons olive oil

Directions:

Take a large skillet pan, place it over medium heat, add oil, and let it heat.

Add eggplant pieces, stir until coated, and then cook for 5 minutes until golden brown.

Add garlic, season with salt and curry powder, cook for 1 minute and then stir in tomatoes.

Cover the skillet pan with its lid and then simmer the vegetables for 7 minutes until thoroughly cooked.

Add potato cubes, drizzle with soy sauce, stir until well combined, and then cook for 1 to 2 minutes until thoroughly hot.

Serve straight away.

Nutritional Information per Serving:

Calories: 76 Cal; Fat: 0.5 g; Protein: 2.5 g; Carbs: 18.3 g; Fiber: 4.4 g;

Lentil Vegetable Curry

Prep Time: 5 minutes; Cooking Time: 25 minutes; Yields: 4 servings;

Ingredients:

2 cups cooked brown rice

1 ½ cup cooked brown lentils

2 cups of frozen mixed vegetables

1 ½ cups diced potatoes

½ cup diced white onion

1 cup diced red bell peppers

2 teaspoons minced garlic

2 dried red peppers, minced

3 tablespoons red curry paste

1 tablespoon olive oil

2 cups coconut milk, unsweetened

Directions:

Take a heatproof bowl, add diced potatoes, and then microwave for 1 minute or until softened.

Place oil in a large pot, place it over medium-high heat and then let it heat until hot.

Add onion, potatoes, and bell pepper, stir in garlic, red pepper, and curry paste and then cook for 10 minutes.

Pour in the milk, continue cooking the curry for 10 minutes until vegetables turn tender, and then stir in lentils.

Cook the curry for 3 minutes until thoroughly hot and then serve.

Nutritional Information per Serving:

Calories: 210 Cal; Fat: 3.2 g; Protein: 12.2 g; Carbs: 35.1 g; Fiber: 13.7 g;

Black Bean Stew

Prep Time: 5 minutes; Cooking Time: 15 minutes; Yields: 6 servings;

Ingredients:

2 green onions, chopped

3 celery, chopped

½ of serrano pepper, chopped

1 teaspoon grated ginger

1 tablespoon lemon zest

2 cups cooked black beans

1 tablespoon olive oil

Directions:

Take a large skillet pan, place it over medium-high heat, add oil and let it heat.

Add black beans, pour in the broth, and then bring it to a boil.

Switch heat to medium level, add onions, celery, ginger, and serrano pepper, stir until mixed, and then cook for 3 to 5 minutes until vegetables are tender-crisp.

Serve the stew with cooked brown rice.

Nutritional Information per Serving:

Calories: 253 Cal; Fat: 5 g; Protein: 32 g; Carbs: 107 g; Fiber: 36 g;

Vegetable Barley Soup

Prep Time: 5 minutes; Cooking Time: 30 minutes; Yields: 6 servings;

Ingredients:

½ cup barley, uncooked

1 cup cauliflower florets

2 medium potatoes, peeled, diced

1 small white onion, peeled, diced

1 cup spinach leaves

2 stalks of celery, diced

1 cup diced carrots

30 ounces fire-roasted tomatoes

1 teaspoon salt

3 tablespoons Creole Seasoning

8 ounces tomato juice

6 cups of water

Directions:

Place a large pot over medium-high heat, add potatoes, cauliflower florets, onion, and barley, pour in the water, and then bring the mixture to a boil.

Add remaining ingredients into the pot except for spinach, stir until combined, and then bring the soup to boil.

Switch heat to medium-low level and then simmer the soup for 20 minutes until vegetables have thoroughly cooked.

When done, stir in spinach, cook for 3 to 5 minutes until leaves wilt and then ladle soup evenly among six bowls.

Serve straight away.

Nutritional Information per Serving:

Calories: 230 Cal; Fat: 4 g; Protein: 11 g; Carbs: 41 g; Fiber: 10 g;

Sweet Potato and Corn Chowder

Prep Time: 5 minutes; Cooking Time: 20 minutes; Yields: 4 servings;

Ingredients:

4 cups canned corn

½ of red onion, peeled, cut into ½-inch cubes

1 medium sweet potato, peeled, cut into ½-inch cubes

1 medium red bell pepper, cored, cut into ½-inch cubes

2 tablespoons minced garlic

½ teaspoon smoked paprika

2 teaspoons avocado oil

1 tablespoon lemon juice

4 cups vegetable broth

2 tablespoons chopped basil

Directions:

Take a large pot, place it over medium heat, add oil, and then let it heat until hot.

Add onion, cook for 2 minutes, stir in garlic and then continue cooking for 1 minute until fragrant.

Add sweet potato and bell pepper pieces, cook for 2 minutes, add corn, stir in paprika and then pour in vegetable stock.

Simmer the vegetables for 15 minutes until tender, then remove the pot from heat and puree the mixture by using an immersion blender until smooth.

Add salt, black pepper, lemon juice, and basil into the chowder, stir until mixed, and then ladle into four bowls.

Serve straight away.

Nutritional Information per Serving:

Calories: 220 Cal; Fat: 3.8 g; Protein: 6.5 g; Carbs: 46.2 g; Fiber: 6.3 g;

Pesto Broccoli Rice

Prep Time: 5 minutes; Cooking Time: 8 minutes; Yields: 6 servings;

Ingredients:

4 cups of broccoli rice

¼ teaspoon salt

¼ teaspoon ground black pepper

¾ cup kale pesto

1 tablespoon olive oil

4 tablespoons grated parmesan cheese

1 lemon, cut into wedges

Directions:

Place a large saucepan over medium heat, add oil and let it heat. .

Add broccoli rice, stir until mixed, and then cook for 4 minutes until tender.

Remove pan from heat, add pesto, stir until mixed, and then remove the pan from heat.

Season with salt and black pepper, add parmesan cheese and then distribute broccoli rice among four bowls.

Serve broccoli rice with a lime wedge.

Nutritional Information per Serving:

Calories: 42 Cal; Fat: 3 g; Protein: 2 g; Carbs: 4 g; Fiber: 2 g;

Pea Soup

Prep Time: 10 minutes; Cooking Time: 1 hour and 20 minutes; Yields: 3 servings;

Ingredients:

1 medium potato, peeled, diced

1 medium carrot, peeled, chopped

½ of a medium white onion, peeled, chopped

1 celery, chopped

½ teaspoon minced garlic

2/3 cup split peas, uncooked

2 tablespoons barley

½ teaspoon salt

1/8 teaspoon dried basil

1/8 teaspoon ground black pepper

1/8 teaspoon dried thyme

1 bay leaf

½ tablespoon olive oil

3 cups of water

2 tablespoons chopped parsley

Directions:

Add oil into a large pot, place it over medium-high heat, and when hot, add onion, garlic, and bay leaf.

Cook for 5 minutes until onion turns soft, add barley and peas, stir in salt, and then pour in water.

Bring the soup to a boil, switch heat to a low level and then simmer the soup for 30 to 50 minutes.

Add remaining ingredients, stir until mixed, and then continue cooking the soup for 15 to 30 minutes until vegetables have cooked.

When done, puree the soup using an immersion blender until smooth, then ladle soup into bowls and then serve.

Nutritional Information per Serving:

Calories: 246.6 Cal; Fat: 2.2 g; Protein: 12.7 g; Carbs: 45.8 g; Fiber: 14.2 g;

Lemon Basil Tofu

Prep Time: 10 minutes; Cooking Time: 10 minutes; Yields: 3 servings;

Ingredients:

16 ounces tofu, pressed, drained

½ of red onion, peeled, sliced

2 teaspoons minced garlic

1 small green bell pepper, cored, sliced

1 tablespoon grated ginger

1 teaspoon maple syrup

3 tablespoons lemon juice

¼ cup of soy sauce

1 tablespoon olive oil

¼ cup basil leaves

Directions:

Cut the tofu into lengthwise slices and then cut each slice into two triangles.

Pour lemon juice into a small bowl, add soy sauce and maple syrup and then stir until mixed.

Place oil in a large frying pan, place it over medium-high heat and when hot, add onion and bell pepper and then cook for 1 minute.

Stir in ginger and garlic, cook for 1 minute, push the vegetables to one side of the pan, add tofu pieces and then cook for 1 minute per side.

Drizzle the soy sauce mixture over tofu pieces, add basil and then continue cooking for 3 minutes per side.

Serve tofu and vegetables with cooked brown rice.

Nutritional Information per Serving:

Calories: 246 Cal; Fat: 3 g; Protein: 12 g; Carbs: 41 g; Fiber: 2 g;

Pumpkin Soup

Prep Time: 5 minutes; Cooking Time: 20 minutes; Yields: 2 servings;

Ingredients:

3 cups pumpkin pieces

¾ teaspoon salt

½ teaspoon ground black pepper

½ teaspoon red chili flakes

2 cups coconut milk, unsweetened

Directions:

Switch on the oven, then set it to 350 degrees F and let it preheat.

Spread the pumpkin pieces on a baking tray, season with salt and black pepper, and then bake for 20 minutes until roasted.

Spoon the pumpkin pieces into a blender, add remaining ingredients and then pulse until smooth.

Distribute the soup evenly among 2 bowls and then serve.

Nutritional Information per Serving:

Calories: 88.6 Cal; Fat: 3.7 g; Protein: 1.8 g; Carbs: 12.4 g; Fiber: 3.8 g;

Broccoli Soup

Prep Time: 5 minutes; Cooking Time: 25 minutes; Yields: 4 bowls;

Ingredients:

15 ounces cooked chickpeas

10 ounces frozen broccoli florets, chopped

6 cups chopped potatoes

1 medium white onion, peeled, diced

1 teaspoon minced garlic

¼ teaspoon ground black pepper

½ tablespoon olive oil

1 lemon, juiced

5 cups vegetable broth

Directions:

Add oil in a medium pan, place it over medium-high heat and let it heat.

Add onion and garlic, cook for 5 minutes until onion begins to tender, and then add potato and broccoli.

Stir in black pepper and lemon juice, pour in the vegetable broth and then bring the soup to a boil.

Switch the heat to medium level, add remaining ingredients and then simmer the soup for 15 minutes until potatoes have cooked and turn tender.

Remove pot from the heat, puree half of the soup using an immersion blender, and stir until combined.

Ladle soup evenly among four bowls and then serve.

Nutritional Information per Serving:

Calories: 87 Cal; Fat: 2 g; Protein: 4 g; Carbs: 14 g; Fiber: 1 g;

Mushroom Steak

Prep Time: 10 minutes; Cooking Time: 45 minutes; Yields: 1 serving;

Ingredients:

1 large oyster mushroom

1/3 teaspoon garlic powder

1 large potato

½ teaspoon salt

4 cherry tomatoes, cut in half

1 tablespoon tahini

½ teaspoon ground black pepper

1 tablespoon chopped parsley

1 tablespoon lemon juice

1 tablespoon water

Directions:

Switch on the oven, then set it to 350 degrees F and let it preheat.

Meanwhile, peel the potato, cut it into strips, drizzle with oil, sprinkle with ¼ teaspoon each of salt and black pepper, and then toss until coated.

Spread potato strips on a baking sheet and then bake for 45 minutes until roasted.

Meanwhile, place a grill pan, place it over medium-high heat, grease it with oil and let it heat.

Season mushrooms with remaining salt and black pepper, place them on the grill pan and then cook for 4 minutes per side until tender. Prepare the sauce and for this, take a small bowl, add parsley, garlic powder, salt, and black pepper, pour in lemon juice and water and then stir in tahini until combined.

When potatoes have roasted, transfer them to a plate, top with mushroom, and then drizzle with prepared sauce.

Serve straight away.

Nutritional Information per Serving:

Calories: 290.9 Cal; Fat: 7.6 g; Protein: 15.2 g; Carbs: 47 g; Fiber: 7.5 g;

Pumpkin Chili

Prep Time: 5 minutes; Cooking Time: 30 minutes; Yields: 4 servings;

Ingredients:

1 cup cooked cannellini beans

1 cup cooked pumpkin

1 cup cooked sweetcorn

1 rib of celery, diced

1 green onion, chopped

1 medium white onion, peeled, sliced

1 jalapeno pepper, chopped

1 medium carrot, peeled, diced

2 cups chopped tomatoes

1 tablespoon minced garlic

1 teaspoon salt

½ teaspoon ground black pepper

1 tablespoon tomato puree

1 cup of water

Directions:

Take a large pot, place it over medium-high heat, add oil, and when hot, add onion and garlic and then cook for 3 minutes until onion turns tender.

Add carrots, celery, and jalapeno, cook the vegetables for 5 minutes, add beans, corn, and pumpkin and then stir in salt and black pepper.

Add tomato, pour in the tomato puree and water, switch heat to medium level and then simmer the chili for 20 minutes until cooked.

Serve straight away.

Nutritional Information per Serving:

Calories: 203.6 Cal; Fat: 1.2 g; Protein: 10.3 g; Carbs: 40.2 g; Fiber: 11.8 g;

Wild Rice Mushroom Soup

Prep Time: 5 minutes; Cooking Time: 40 minutes; Yields: 4;

Ingredients:

½ cup chopped white onion

8 ounces cremini mushrooms, sliced

1 jalapeño, chopped

1 tablespoon minced garlic

1 cup wild rice blend

1 teaspoon taco seasoning

½ teaspoon ground black pepper

¾ teaspoon salt

½ teaspoon red pepper flakes

1 teaspoon poultry seasoning

½ teaspoon dried thyme

2 teaspoons olive oil

½ cup cashew cream

4 cups of water

½ cup of salsa

Directions:

Switch on the instant pot, press the sauté button, add oil into the inner pot and then let it heat.

Add onion, mushrooms, jalapeno, and garlic, and then cook for 3 minutes until vegetable begin to soften.

Add rice and salsa, stir in salt and all the spices and herbs until well mixed, press the cancel button, and then shut the instant pot with its lid.

Press the manual button, cook at high pressure for 30 minutes, and when the instant pot beeps, do a natural pressure release.

Stir the soup, add cashew cream, stir until well mixed, press the sauté button and then bring the soup to boil until thoroughly hot.

Taste the soup to adjust seasoning and then serve.

Nutritional Information per Serving:

Calories: 274 Cal; Fat: 11 g; Protein: 10 g; Carbs: 38 g; Fiber: 5 g;

Lentil with Spinach

Prep Time: 5 minutes; Cooking Time: 25 minutes; Yields: 2;

Ingredients:

½ cup red lentils

1 cup chopped spinach

½ teaspoon mustard seeds

½ teaspoon ground turmeric

1/3 teaspoon cumin seeds

1/3 teaspoon cayenne

1/3 teaspoon nigella seeds

2/3 teaspoon salt

1/8 teaspoon fennel seeds

1/8 teaspoon fenugreek seeds

1 teaspoon olive oil

2 ½ cups water

Directions:

Take a large saucepan, place it over medium heat, add oil and then let it heat until hot.

Add all the seeds, stir until coated in oil, and then cook for 1 to 2 minutes until seeds begin to pop.

Stir in cayenne pepper and turmeric, stir in lentils and then cook for 1 minute until roasted.

Season with salt, pour in the water, and then cook for 20 minutes until lentils have thoroughly cooked; cover the pan partially with its lid.

Stir in spinach, simmer for 2 minutes until spinach leaves wilts, and then serve.

Nutritional Information per Serving:

Calories: 193 Cal; Fat: 3 g; Protein: 12 g; Carbs: 28 g; Fiber: 14 g;

Carrots and Quinoa Veggie Bowl

Prep Time: 10 minutes; Cooking Time: 0 minutes; Yields: 3;

Ingredients:

2/3 cup quinoa

7 kale leaves, de-stemmed, chopped

2 cups cooked chickpeas

2 carrots, spiralized

½ of an orange, peeled, sliced

2 green onions, sliced

1 large avocado, peeled, pitted, sliced

1 cup chopped parsley

½ teaspoon salt

½ teaspoon ground black pepper

2 tablespoons toasted walnuts, crushed

½ of a lemon, juiced

Directions:

Prepare the quinoa, and for this, cook by following the instruction on its package and, when done, fluff it with a fork and set aside until required.

Meanwhile, place chopped kale leaves in a large, drizzle with lemon juice, sprinkle with some salt and black pepper, and then massage for 1 minute.

Scatter kale leaves evenly among three plates, top with chickpeas, quinoa, carrots, and parsley, season with salt and black pepper, and then drizzle with lemon juice.

Scatter orange and avocado slices evenly on top of the salad, sprinkle with walnuts and then serve.

Nutritional Information per Serving:

Calories: 306 Cal; Fat: 21 g; Protein: 21 g; Carbs: 68 g; Fiber: 23 g;

Dessert Recipes

Chocolate and Avocado Pudding

Prep Time: 5 minutes; Cooking Time: 15 minutes; Yields: 2 servings;

Ingredients:

2 medium avocados

1 teaspoon shredded coconut

½ teaspoon salt

1 tablespoon coconut sugar

2 ½ tablespoons cocoa powder

1 tablespoon maple syrup

1 ½ tablespoon almond milk, unsweetened

Directions:

Place all the ingredients except for coconut in the jar of a blender or food processor and then pulse until smooth.

Spoon the pudding into a bowl, sprinkle coconut on top and then serve.

Nutritional Information per Serving:

Calories: 267.5 Cal; Fat: 13.5 g; Protein: 1.8 g; Carbs: 8.7 g; Fiber: 6 g;

Chocolate Covered Dates

Prep Time: 1 hour and 10 minutes; Cooking Time: 3 minutes; Yields: 16;

Ingredients:

16 Medjool dates, pitted

½ teaspoon of sea salt

¾ cup almonds

1 teaspoon coconut oil

8 ounces chocolate chips

Directions:

Take a medium baking sheet, line it with parchment paper, and then set aside until required.

Place an almond into the pit of each date and then wrap the date tightly around it.

Place chocolate chips in a heatproof bowl, add oil, and then microwave for 2 to 3 minutes until chocolate melts, stirring every minute.

Working on one date at a time, dip each date into the chocolate mixture and then place it onto the prepared baking sheet.

Sprinkle salt over the prepared dates and then let them rest in the refrigerator for 1 hour until chocolate is firm.

Serve straight away.

Nutritional Information per Serving:

Calories: 179 Cal; Fat: 7.7 g; Protein: 3 g; Carbs: 28.5 g; Fiber: 3 g;

Chocolate Chip Cookies

Prep Time: 10 minutes; Cooking Time: 10 minutes; Yields: 6 servings;

Ingredients:

2 ½ cups white whole-wheat flour

1 teaspoon baking soda

½ cup of coconut sugar

½ teaspoon salt

2 teaspoons vanilla extract, unsweetened

¼ cup brown sugar

½ cup coconut butter

1 cup dark chocolate chip

¼ cup olive oil

¼ cup of water

Directions:

Switch on the oven, then set it to 375 degrees F and let it preheat.

Take a large baking sheet, line it with parchment paper, and then set aside until required.

Place sugar in a large bowl, add vanilla, oil, butter, and water, and then blend by using an immersion blender until well combined.

Blend in salt, baking soda, and flour until incorporated and then fold in chocolate chips.

Scoop the prepared dough on the baking sheet using an ice cream scoop, flatten each cookie slightly by using a spatula and then bake for 10 minutes until cookies turn crisp and golden brown • around the edges. When done, let cookies cool completely and then serve.

Nutritional Information per Serving:

Calories: 180 Cal; Fat: 10 g; Protein: 2 g; Carbs: 19 g; Fiber: 2 g;

Pumpkin and Chocolate Brownies

Prep Time: 10 minutes; Cooking Time: 25 minutes; Yields: 16 brownies;

Ingredients:

1 ¼ cup white whole-wheat flour

½ teaspoon salt

2 teaspoons baking powder

½ cup of cocoa powder

1/3 cup maple syrup

¼ cup olive oil

1 ½ cup pumpkin puree

Directions:

Switch on the oven, then set it to 350 degrees F and let it preheat.

Meanwhile, take a large bowl, place all the ingredients in it and then whisk until smooth.

Take a 9-by-9 inch baking pan, grease it with oil, spoon the batter in it and then bake for 25 minutes until almost set.

When done, remove the pan from the oven and then let the brownie cool completely.

Then cut the brownie into squares and serve.

Nutritional Information per Serving:

Calories: 122 Cal; Fat: 2 g; Protein: 2 g; Carbs: 25 g; Fiber: 6 g;

Chocolate Bark

Prep Time: 10 minutes; Cooking Time: 35 minutes; Yields: 8 pieces;

Ingredients:

15 ounces cooked chickpeas

1/8 teaspoon sea salt

1 cup dark chocolate chips

1 tablespoon olive oil

Directions:

Switch on the oven, then set it to 400 degrees F and let it preheat.

Pat dry the chickpeas, place them in a bowl, add oil and then toss until coated.

Spread the chickpeas on a baking sheet, sprinkle with salt and then bake for 30 minutes until chickpeas turn golden brown, stirring every 10 minutes.

Then remove the baking sheet from the oven and let them cool completely.

Meanwhile, place the chocolate chips in a heatproof bowl and then microwave for 1 to 2 minutes at a high heat setting until chocolate melts, stirring every 30 seconds.

When the chickpeas are cooled, add chickpeas into the melted chocolate, and then toss until coated.

Spread the chickpeas evenly on the baking sheet and then let it cool until firm.

Cut the chickpeas and chocolate into eight pieces and then serve. .

Nutritional Information per Serving:

Calories: 158 Cal; Fat: 9.8 g; Protein: 0.4 g; Carbs: 20.5 g; Fiber: 2.3 g;

Strawberry and Banana Ice Cream

Prep Time: 5 minutes; Cooking Time: 0 minutes; Yields: 2 servings;

Ingredients:

3 cups sliced and frozen bananas

1 tablespoon maple syrup

½ teaspoon vanilla extract, unsweetened

- 1 cup strawberries, fresh

Directions:

Place all the ingredients in the jar of a blender or food processor and then pulse until smooth.

Divide the ice cream between two bowls and then serve.

Nutritional Information per Serving:

Calories: 166 Cal; Fat: 6 g; Protein: 1 g; Carbs: 30 g; Fiber: 4 g;

No-Bake Chocolate Pie

Prep Time: 6 hours and 10 minutes; Cooking Time: 0 minutes; Yields: 6 slices;

Ingredients:

1 prepared crust of pie

2/3 cup chocolate chips, melted

For the Filling:

1 pound of silken tofu

½ teaspoon salt

1 teaspoon vanilla extract, unsweetened

3 tablespoons maple syrup

1 cup coconut milk, unsweetened

Directions:

Prepare the filling and for this, place all of its ingredients in a large bowl and then blend until smooth.

Reserve 1 cup of the filling mixture, place it in a medium bowl, add the melted chocolate and then stir until combined.

Place the crust in a pie pan, spoon chocolate filling it, then top with the reserved filling and make designs using a butter knife.

Place the pie into the refrigerator and then chill it for 4 to 6 hours in the refrigerator until firm.

Cut the pie into slices and then serve.

Nutritional Information per Serving:

Calories: 304.3 Cal; Fat: 15.4 g; Protein: 6.6 g; Carbs: 37.6 g; Fiber: 1.3 g;

Fudge Brownies

Prep Time: 10 minutes; Cooking Time: 30 minutes; Yields: 9 brownies;

Ingredients:

1 cup white whole-wheat flour

½ teaspoon baking powder

¾ cup of sugar

¾ cup chocolate chips

6 tablespoons cocoa powder

¼ teaspoon salt

1 teaspoon vanilla extract, unsweetened

2 tablespoons coconut oil

½ cup of water

½ cup applesauce, unsweetened

Directions:

Switch on the oven, then set it to 350 degrees F and let it preheat.

Take a large bowl, pour in water and applesauce, add oil and vanilla and then whisk until combined.

Take a separate large bowl, add remaining ingredients in it except for chocolate chips and then stir until mixed.

Stir the flour mixture into the applesauce mixture, 4 tablespoons at a time, until incorporated.

Take a square casserole dish, grease it with oil, spoon the batter in it and then sprinkle chocolate chips on top.

Bake the brownie for 30 minutes until almost set and then let it cool. .

Cut the brownie into squares and then serve.

Nutritional Information per Serving:

Calories: 280 Cal; Fat: 14 g; Protein: 3 g; Carbs: 40 g; Fiber: 2 g;

Caramel Slice

Prep Time: 1 hour; Cooking Time: 0 minutes; Yields: 6 slices;

Ingredients:

For the Base:

¼ cup of cocoa powder

½ cup almonds

½ cup Medjool dates pitted

2 tablespoons melted coconut oil

For the Caramel Layer:

2 tablespoons maple syrup

1 cup Medjool dates, pitted

4 tablespoons tahini pasta

½ cup melted coconut oil

1 teaspoon vanilla extract, unsweetened

For the Chocolate Layer:

¼ cup maple syrup

¼ cup of cocoa powder

¼ cup melted coconut oil

Directions:

Prepare the base and for this, place all of its ingredients in a blender or food processor and then pulse until sticky crumble mixture comes together.

Take a square dish, spoon the base mixture in it, spread it evenly, and then let it rest in the freezer until required.

Prepare the caramel and for this, place all of its ingredients in a blender and then pulse until smooth.

Spread the caramel mixture over the base and then let it rest for 30 minutes in the freezer.

Prepare the chocolate layer and for this, place all of its ingredients in a medium bowl and then whisk until combined.

Pour the chocolate mixture over the caramel layer, spread evenly, and then let it rest for 10 minutes in the freezer.

When ready to eat, let the caramel slice rest for 10 minutes at room temperature, then cut it into slices and then serve.

Nutritional Information per Serving:

Calories: 60 Cal; Fat: 2.6 g; Protein: 0.5 g; Carbs: 7.4 g; Fiber: 1.4 g;

Creamsicles

Prep Time: 4 hours and 5 minutes; Cooking Time: 0 minutes; Yields: 5;

Ingredients:

3 tablespoons agave syrup

1 cup coconut milk, unsweetened

½ teaspoon vanilla extract, unsweetened

1 cup of orange juice

Directions:

Place all the ingredients in a food processor or blender and then pulse until combined.

Pour the mixture into five molds of Popsicle pan, insert a stick into each mold and then let it freeze for a minimum of 4 hours until hard.

Serve when ready.

Nutritional Information per Serving:

Calories: 152 Cal; Fat: 10 g; Protein: 1 g; Carbs: 16 g; Fiber: 1 g;

No-Bake Cookies

Prep Time: 30 minutes; Cooking Time: 0 minutes; Yields: 9;

Ingredients:

1 cup rolled oats

¼ cup of cocoa powder

1/8 teaspoon salt

1 teaspoon vanilla extract, unsweetened

¼ cup and 2 tablespoons peanut butter, divided

6 tablespoons coconut oil, divided

¼ cup and 1 tablespoon maple syrup, divided

Directions:

Take a small saucepan, place it over low heat, add 5 tablespoons of coconut oil and then let it melt.

Whisk in 2 tablespoons peanut butter, salt, 1 teaspoon vanilla extract, and ¼ cup each of cocoa powder and maple syrup, and then whisk until well combined.

Remove pan from heat, stir in oats and then spoon the mixture evenly into 9 cups of a muffin pan.

Wipe clean the pan, return it over low heat, add remaining coconut oil, maple syrup, and peanut butter, stir until combined, and then cook for 2 minutes until thoroughly warmed.

Drizzle the peanut butter sauce over the oat mixture in the muffin pan and then let it freeze for 20 minutes or more until set.

Serve straight away.

Nutritional Information per Serving:

Calories: 213 Cal; Fat: 14.8 g; Protein: 4 g; Carbs: 17.3 g; Fiber: 2.1 g;

Chocolate Strawberry Shake

Prep Time: 5 minutes; Cooking Time: 0 minutes; Yields: 2;

Ingredients:

2 cups almond milk, unsweetened

4 bananas, peeled, frozen

4 tablespoons cocoa powder

2 cups strawberries, frozen

Directions:

Place all the ingredients into the jar of a high-speed food processor or blender in the order stated in the ingredients list and then cover it with the lid.

Pulse for 1 minute until smooth, and then serve.

Nutritional Information per Serving:

Calories: 208 Cal; Fat: 0.2 g; Protein: 12.4 g; Carbs: 26.2 g; Fiber: 1.4 g;

Chocolate Clusters

Prep Time: 15 minutes; Cooking Time: 0 minutes; Yields: 24;

Ingredients:

1 cup chopped dark chocolate

1 cup cashews, roasted, salt

1 teaspoon sea salt flakes

Directions:

Take a large baking sheet, line it with wax paper, and then set aside until required.

Take a medium bowl, place chocolate in it, and then microwave for 1 minute.

Stir the chocolate and then continue microwaving it at 1-minute intervals until chocolate melts completely, stirring at every interval.

When melted, stir the chocolate to bring it to 90 degrees F and then stir in cashews.

Scoop the walnut-chocolate mixture on the prepared baking sheet, ½ tablespoons per cluster, and then sprinkle with salt.

Let the clusters stand at room temperature until harden and then serve.

Nutritional Information per Serving:

Calories: 79.4 Cal; Fat: 6.6 g; Protein: 1 g; Carbs: 5.8 g; Fiber: 1.1 g;

Chocolate Pots

Prep Time: 4 hours and 10 minutes; Cooking Time: 3 minutes; Yields: 4;

Ingredients:

6 ounces chocolate, unsweetened

1 cup Medjool dates, pitted

1 ¾ cups almond milk, unsweetened

Directions:

Cut the chocolate into small pieces, place them in a heatproof bowl and then microwave for 2 to 3 minutes until melt completely, stirring every minute.

Place dates in a blender, pour in the milk, and then pulse until smooth.

Add chocolate into the blender and then pulse until combined.

Divide the mixture into the small mason jars and then let them rest for 4 hours until set.

Serve straight away.

Nutritional Information per Serving:

Calories: 321 Cal; Fat: 19 g; Protein: 6 g; Carbs: 34 g; Fiber: 4 g;

Maple and Tahini Fudge

Prep Time: 1 hour and 100 minutes; Cooking Time: 3 minutes; Yields: 15;

Ingredients:

1 cup dark chocolate chips

¼ cup maple syrup

½ cup tahini

Directions:

Take a heatproof bowl, place chocolate chips in it and then microwave for 2 to 3 minutes until melt completely, stirring every minute.

When melted, remove the chocolate bowl from the oven and then whisk in maple syrup and tahini until smooth.

Take a 4-by-8 inches baking dish, line it with wax paper, spoon the chocolate mixture in it and then press it into the baking dish.

Cover with another sheet with wax paper, press it down until smooth, and then let the fudge rest for 1 hour in the freezer until set.

Then cut the fudge into 15 squares and serve.

Nutritional Information per Serving:

Calories: 110.7 Cal; Fat: 5.3 g; Protein: 2.2 g; Carbs: 15.1 g; Fiber: 1.6 g;

Conclusion

And that is everything you need to know about the Sirtfood Diet. To tell the truth, the study into sirtuin is relatively new, and therefore, we still know quite little about it.

Keep in mind that we are all different. Two people following the same diet to a T would still get different results. Therefore, do not be disheartened if the Sirtfood Diet does not work for you. But if you are unsure whether you should try it, we highly recommend you give it a shot. Many celebrities tried it, and it worked well for them. It is worth giving it a shot if you've tried out many other diet regimens, and none of them worked for you.

Finally, make sure you listen to your body. If you start to experience any more serious symptoms other than what has been described above, then perhaps your body does not respond well to the diet. Then, you are advised to change your diet and move on to something else.

The Sirtfood Diet is intended to be a lifestyle change, not a one-time diet. It encourages people to start living a healthy life, starting with the introduction of healthy food. If you cannot follow the Sirtfood Diet, you can still lose at least a pound or two just by exercising and eating plant-based food or cut out processed food from your life.

With all that said and done, we wish you the very best in your journey toward health and fitness.

Italian Cookbook

Ciao! Food is Italy, and Italy is food!

Have you always been a *foodie* who has a tangible passion for authentic and classic Italian cooking? Then this book is for you.

It will take you on a culinary journey through the 20 regions of Italy, with a 'stopover' in each region, where you will find dishes akin to the area.

The recipes are easy to follow and understand. It comes complete with wine pairing suggestions and even a few Italian terms to learn and enjoy.

Embrace your inner Italian and explore all this comprehensive book offers with beautiful images scattered throughout the cookbook.

The recipes that you will find in here provide all the ingredients as well as easy to follow step-by-step instructions on how to achieve perfection!

If you like the book, don't hesitate to tell me your opinion, it is very important to me, I wish you a good reading!

Table of Contents

Introduction: Iconic Italian Genealogy 1

The 20 Regions of Italy 2

The Five Autonomous Regions of Italy............................2

Friuli-Venezia Giulia 2

Sardinia 3

Sicily 3

Trentino-Alto Adige 4

Val D'Aosta 4

The Other 15 Regions of Italy 5

Abruzzo 5

Apulia (Puglia) 5

Basilicata 6

Calabria 6

Campania 7

Emilia-Romagna 8

Lazio 8

Liguria 9

Lombardy 9

Marche 10

Molise..10

Piedmont...10

Tuscany 11

Umbria 11

Veneto 12

Agriculture, Livestock, Fisheries, Forestry, and More 12

Agriculture 12

Livestock 13

Fisheries 13

Forestry...14

Hunting..14

How Italian Food Took the World by Storm..................14

The Italian Kitchen Icon: aka Nonna!.........................15

Products of Genuine Italian Origin.............................16

The Essential Pantry Staples for Italian Cooking..........18

Chapter 1: Perfect Antipasti **20**

The Italian Ham Selection.......................................20

Antipasti Recipes You Can Try at Home......................22

    Taralli Le Puglia..22

    Parma Ham Pockets With Asparagus and Peas 23

    Pepperoni all'Acciuga 25

    Fregola Salad 26

    Prosciutto Crudo & Leek Involtini........................27

Chapter 2: Pasta Dishes **30**

Characteristics of Quality, Authentic Pasta.................30

Types of Italian Pasta 31

Why You Should Invest in an Italian Pasta Maker 32

Some Renowned Pasta Makers 33

Basic Italian Pasta Dough Recipe..............................33

Pasta Recipes for You to Try at Home.........................34

    Cjalsons (Cjarsons) 34

    Pasta alla Norma...36

    Anelli alla Pecoraro..38

    Bucatini all'amatriciana.....................................41

    Spaghetti alla Marchigiana 42

    Agnolotti del Plin 44

Chapter 3: Meat, Poultry, and Salumi 47

Beef..47

    Bresaola 47

    Veal 47

Poultry 47

   Chicken...47

   Duck 48

   Goose 48

Pork.. 48

   Guanciale... 48

   Lardo 49

   Pancetta.. 49

   Pork 49

   Prosciutto 49

   Salumi 49

   Sausage... 49

   Lamb 50

   Venison/Game 50

Moreish Meat, Poultry, and Salumi Recipes 50

   Goulash Triestino.. 50

   Smacafam..52

   Lasagna Valdostana 53

   Saltimbocca 55

   Pampanella Molisana...56

Chapter 4: Italian Fish Cuisine.................... 58

Feast of the Seven Fishes.. 58

   Fregola allo Scoglio 59

   Brodetto alla Vastese... 60

   Risotto alla Pescatora... 62

   Lumache alla Bresciana 63

   Bagna cauda 65

   Whitebait With Dill Mayonnaise 66

Chapter 5: Rice Dishes for the Win 68

Rice Is Born in Water and Must Die in Wine 68

   Risotto ai Mirtilli e Speck....................................... 68

Italian Wild Rice Soup..70

Piedmontese Carnaroli Risotto With Veal Tongue, Hazelnuts, and Grana Padano 71

Risotto Primavera 73

Chapter 6: Vegetarian Dishes..**75**

Wholesome Vegetarian Recipes 76

Fave e Cicoria..76

Erbazzone 77

Frittata Rafano e Pecorino..79

Parmigiana Stacks 80

Chapter 7: Italian Bread.. **82**

Italian Bread Recipes..82

Gnocchi di Pane Raffermo..84

Homemade Veneto Ciabatta Bread 86

Crescia Sfogliata..87

Tuscan Panzanella Salad 88

Chapter 8: Desserts.. **90**

Delicious Italian Desserts..90

Pressnitz..90

Cannoli Siciliani..92

Torta con le Mele 94

Pasticioto 95

Tartufo 97

Caragnoli..99

Conclusion **101**

Italian Cooking A Glossary of Terms **103**

Italian Folk Sayings Translated.. **107**

References **115**

Introduction: Iconic Italian Genealogy

Ciao tutti! Italian heritage is one of the most culture-rich civilizations to date, from its deep roots in the diverse blend of epochal societies such as the Romans and the Samnites, straight through to embracing non-native peoples such as the Greeks and Phoenicians.

Proudly dubbed the birthplace of opera, Italy has many offerings to afford her natives and any visitors. She is famous for cultural components such as:

- Amazing food
- Music
- Renaissance art
- Style

The layout of this beautiful country is intricately shaped to resemble a boot and boasts several world-renowned cities. This country is probably the most famous for its cuisine and its proud people.

The 20 Regions of Italy

Italy is subdivided into 20 different regions, resembling states or provinces—as they are called in other countries. With so many unique characteristics, it can be hard for a first-time traveler to fit in all of the fantastic activities and sights on offer unless you plan to take a trip and just explore Italy on its own.

There are 20 regions in total, of which five are autonomous. Autonomous means that they have a broader sense of freedom in terms of finances, politics, etc. The word autonomy, in itself, means to have a sense of self-governance.

The Five Autonomous Regions of Italy

Friuli-Venezia Giulia

This is one of the smaller regions, located on the northeast side of the country. Don't be fooled by its size, as it offers both dazzling seaside views and mountains that border the Alps. If you fancy yourself both sea and hills during your vacation, then this is, without a doubt, one of the regions to visit on your Italian bucket list.

Fact: According to popular folklore, Friuli was once home to a covenant of wizards, sorcerers, and magicians that performed rituals and other magic such as exorcisms circa the 16th and 17th centuries.

These druids and spellcasters reportedly practiced both good and bad magic, and were summoned to court and sentenced for dabbling in enchantments.

Traditional Food: *Paparot, Strucchi, Tiramisu.*

Sardinia

Planning a trip outside of July and August will afford each visitor the tranquil beach settings that this region offers. On the flip side of the coin, this is an excellent spot for a bit of clubbing and other nocturnal social activities.

Fact: It is said that people from Sardinia have the longest life expectancy in the world. Inhabitants are known to reach considerable centenary numbers in age, with 22 people out of every 100 000 inhabitants. It makes you wonder what their secret is. Is there a mystery that is hidden from the rest of the world?

Traditional Food: *Zuppa Gallurese, Bottarga, Seadas*

Sicily

Sicily is the largest region in Italy and also possesses bragging rights when it comes to the region with the best ancient ruins in the whole of Italy.

Challenge yourself and plan a climbing expedition to Mount Etna, which is the biggest active volcano on the European continent.

Fact: Due to the charm and beauty that this region has to present, it is no wonder that it became a preferred filming location for several well-known movies centered around the *Mob Italiano*! The most famous of these has to be *The Godfather Trilogy*, which was filmed in 1972, 1974, and 1990 by none other than Francis Ford Coppola.

Traditional Food: *Arancini, Caponata, Raw Red Prawns*

Trentino-Alto Adige

How about combining a bit of German and Italian at the same time, while only visiting one country? Yes, this is indeed possible! This region formed part of Austria-Hungary since it came into existence and was only seized by Italy in 1919. Interestingly enough, the majority of its people speak German, as opposed to Italian.

Fact: This region is laden with wall upon wall of jagged dolomite. The Dolomite mountain ranges were added to the UNESCO World Natural Heritage list in 2009. The basis of the addition to this exclusive club is attributed to the fact that the formation of this type of limestone started around 250 million years ago as a coral reef underneath the Tethys Ocean.

Traditional Food: *Kaiserschmarren, Canederli, Schiacciatina*

Val D'Aosta

This region is located in Northwest Italy and borders Switzerland and France. It has not one but two medieval castles, making it one of the wealthiest areas in all of Italy. The Courmayeur resort on Mont Blanc that is situated in the Aosta Valley is one of the most fabulous resorts in Europe, frequented as the playground of the rich and famous.

Fact: Although the smallest region in Italy, it boasts a wide range of cultural games and sports. One such example is that of *Fiolet*. *Fiolet* can be practiced both as a team or as an individual sport. The aim of the sport is to bounce an oval-shaped ball resembling an egg (fiolet) off a smooth stone with a wooden mallet. The game is won by the person that hits it the furthest while it is still suspended in the air.

Traditional Food: *Polenta Concia, Vapelenentse Soup, Valdostana Ribs*

The Other 15 Regions of Italy

Abruzzo

Due to the rural location of this scenic region, it is not visited often. Apart from the quaint landscapes, it creates the perfect balance year round, with sunny beaches in summer and crisp, white mountains blanketed with snow in the winter. Many visitors are disheartened to visit this region, due to its poverty-stricken status. It had made a remarkable recovery but suffered a catastrophic blow in 2009 when its capital, L'Aquila, was hit by a massive earthquake.

Fact: It is one of the least population-dense regions in Italy and ranked seventh on the list of Italian regions when it comes to a citizen headcount. There is another significant advantage to this region for oenophiles (wine lovers), Abruzzo has a free red wine fountain. Yes, you can travel and stop for a glass of quality Italian wine on your journey! What about this does not sound great? Right?

Traditional Food: *Pizzelle, Fiadoni, Imballo Abruzzese*

Apulia (Puglia)

The best time of year to visit this tourist-popular region is spring or autumn, as the high summer temperatures might be unbearable to some travelers.

Puglia is located in the heel of the Italian boot, as seen on a world map.

Fact: The name Puglia is pronounced as *poo-li-ya* and it is responsible for producing 40% of the country's olive oil demand.

Traditional Food: *Fave e Cicoria, Rustico, Panzerotti*

Basilicata

The region of Basilicata has one of the shortest coastlines in Italy and is located on the instep of the famous boot. It is nestled between Calabria and Puglia and its capital is Potenza. One of its greatest tourist attractions has to be the Neolithic cave dwellings in Matera—which are also a World Heritage Site. **Fact:** This region is sometimes overlooked, but a lesser-known fact is that it has a special cultivar of wine called *Aglianicodel Vulture.* This wine has been awarded the highest appellation by the *Denominazione di origine controllata e garantita* (DOCG). This is the highest tier of wine that can be achieved in the Italian wine classification order.

Traditional Food: *Basilicata, Matera Bread, Rafanata*

Calabria

This region forms part of the toe of the Italian *stivale*, with its capital being Catanzaro. Calabria is excellent for a remote hideaway, focused on hiking in the splendor of her four mountain ranges.

Fact: During events and special occasions, the *Calabria Tarantella* is played, and pairs of men and women dressed in brightly colored costumes of red,
green, and white (yes, to honor the Italian flag) feverishly dance to this upbeat and well-known tune. Traditionally, the Tarantella was assumed to be a cure for a tarantula spider bite. It was believed that you could cure yourself of the poison injected by the spider's venom by sweating it out. Today, it is used as a form of seduction when luring a partner... much like some arachnids.

Traditional Food: *Zuppuli, Ginetti, Tartufo*

Campania

Campania is one of the culturally rich regions of Italy. It is densely populated and has five provinces in its confines. The biggest draw to tourists when it comes to this region is the Amalfi Coast. The Greek ruins of Paestum is also a must-see for any archaeological enthusiast.

Fact: The inspiration behind the 1812 ballet *Il Noce di Benevento* is based on an old Italian myth of Benevento's witches from the same region. The tale says that Beneveto became a place of gathering for hexes to meet under a walnut tree. During the day, they disguised themselves and walked among the people, but at night they would confer and chant a terribly evil spell reported to cause horrific events such as miscarriages and abortions to those they cursed.

Traditional Food: *Parmigiana Melanzane, Polpette, Fritto Misto di Mare*

Emilia-Romagna

There are so many wonderful reasons to visit this opulent region, from the F1 motor racing event at the Imola circuit, to the multitude of castles, and not to mention the flavorsome Modena balsamic vinegar and Parmigiano-Reggiano cheese. If, for no other reason, visit it for the culinary experiences you can indulge in.

Fact: Emilia-Romagna is home to some of Italy's most famed car manufacturers. The list comprises names such as Ferrari, Maserati, and Lamborghini. Be still my beating heart!

Traditional Food: *Borgotaro malfatti, Bolognese Ragú, Erbazzone*

Lazio

This is the third most population dense region in Italy and is home to Rome! With so many historical sites to visit, such as the Vatican, Gaeta, Anzio, Tivoli, Ostia, and Palatine hills, you definitely won't be disappointed if this is your thing. If you fancy yourself a bit of a botanist, you can also visit a Renaissance garden or two.

Fact: Nearly €700 000 coins are tossed into the Trevi Fountain annually. The money is then donated to Caritas to help the poor.

Traditional Food: *Carciofi alla Romana, Quinto Quarto, Puntarelle alla Romana*

Liguria

When visiting this region, you can expect to encounter other exciting sites such as Monaco, Cannes, and San Marino along the way. This region was also home to the famous seafarer Christopher Colombus.

Fact: This region is also known as the Italian Riviera. One of Italy's most famous sauces, pesto, calls Liguria its birthplace.

Traditional Food: *Burrida, Pandolce, Trofie*

Lombardy

Lombardy can brag with a capital that is the home of Italian fashion and extravagant nightlife. This is none other than Milan. One of the other big crowd-pullers that attracts tourists to this region is the expanse of lakes Como and Garda.

The Autodromo Nazionale Monza is also located in this incredible region. It is home to many an Italian Formula 1 race. Native Italian-American son, Mario Andretti, clinched the F1 Driver's World Championship at this very circuit in 1977.

Fact: Happy hour in Milan is an indulgent occurrence, with patrons consuming bitter *aperitivos*, that are mixed into cocktails such as Campari and Negroni. Drink o'clock in this region is simply *la dolce vita*!

Traditional Food: *Cotoletta alla Milanese, Pumpkin Tortelli, Panettone*

Marche

This hidden region produces many of Italy's furniture and textiles. Tourists who have visited this region, prefer it for the quiet, sandy beaches and the R and R that accompanies it.

Fact: Marche has been the official shoe-producing capital of Italy since the 1960s. It is split into three shoe-making repositories that see each repo making a different specialized shoe type. Being Italian and all, there is even a Footwear Museum to visit.

Traditional Food: *Moscioli, Olive all'ascolana, Ciausculo*

Molise

This is the newest addition to the list of regions in Italy and is small in scale. Primarily this region is a cultivator of a range of agricultural products such as wine and cereals.

Fact: Molise produces meat and is therefore ideal to visit, if you are looking at experiencing lip-smackingly good Italian food such as *pampanella* and *pezzata*.

Traditional Food: *Composta Molisana, Caciocavallo di Agnone, Cauciuni*

Piedmont

Another item on the Italian to-visit list for foodies! With its slow food organization—meaning the promotion of local food and authentic cooking—you can expect classical Italian dishes from breakfast to dinner.

Fact: Approximately 170 000 acres of the Piedmont region is made up of vineyards. Therefore it comes as no surprise that this region is renowned for some esteemed Italian wine labels.

Traditional Food: *Agnolotti del Plin, Bagna Cauda (also Bagna Caôda), Carne Cruda all'albese*

Tuscany

The Italian Renaissance period is said to have originated in Tuscany as is the Italian language as we know it today. Due to its reputation, this region can be perceived as somewhat mainstream and can be overcrowded at the best of times. Not to mention that it is quite pricey.

Fact: Tuscany was the first European region to adopt sidewalks or pavements as they are more commonly known. The city of Florence became a pioneer of this occurrence in 1339, and soon the rest of Europe followed suit.

Traditional Food: *Torta di Ceci, Aquacotta, Lampredotto*

Umbria

This region is found in the center of the Italian boot. It is the neighboring region of Tuscany and thus is regularly compared to its counterpart.

Fact: A fact that will excite tourists is that underneath the city, a network of tunnels and grottos can be found and explored. During World War II, this tunneling system served as a bomb shelter to its occupants.

Traditional Food: *Lumachine alle Schegginese, Brustengolo, Porchetta*

Veneto

The region of Veneto is very well known across the world for its capital city, Venice. It is one of the Italian regions that boasts the largest number of tourists per year (in excess of 60 million). The intricate canal system, carnivals, and gothic architecture make this a unique part of Italy.

Fact: There are only 400 licensed gondolas in the Venetian fleet, and to become a gondolier is harder than it appears on the surface. Lengthy onboarding and training sessions have to be passed, as well as a history test of Venice, before a gondoliere is issued with a license to drive...or is it steer?

Traditional Food: *Risi e Bisi, Polenta e Uccelli, Pastissada de Caval*

Agriculture, Livestock, Fisheries, Forestry, and More

Agriculture

Italy has subdivided its agriculture into four categories, namely:

- Field crops
- Forestry
- Pastures
- Tree crops

This country is a crucial rice exporter. Both rice and corn are primarily grown on the Po plain. Second to rice, tomatoes are the next major component produced for exportation, with Naples and Emilia-Romagna yielding the most prominent crops.

Livestock

It is estimated that 10 749 000 acres in Italy consist of pasture and meadows. Inadequate national production forced Italy to import substantial amounts of corn. According to researchers, animal husbandry in 2001 yielded 4 141 000 tons of meat that year (Animal husbandry - Italy - import, farming, n.d.). The production was a culmination of hogs, cattle, sheep, and goats.

Even though Italy has a good production rate, the dairy market is still much underdeveloped today.

Fisheries

In the last four decades of the 20th century, the fish production in Italy increased to almost double. However, the 21st century saw exactly the opposite happen. Between 1998 and 2010, wild fish species were mainly caught in the Mediterranean.

The birth of the aquaculture concept, where species such as algae, aquatic plants, mollusks, fish, and crustaceans from both fresh and saltwater environments are cultivated together and regulated by a controlled environment, has had a notable impact on the fishing sector.

Forestry

Forestry in Italy is primarily made up of trees with broad leaves, whereby conifers, in particular, make up a fifth of the numbers in total. The conifer fauna is predominantly found at the Alpine foothills in Trentino-Alto Adige.

Unfortunately, due to the forests' overutilization by the Romans and other civilizations in the 19th century, there is not much woodland left in Italy. This is mainly due to the wood being used to create items such as mine shafts and railway sleepers, amongst others.

Hunting

Hunting is an all-year activity in Italy. Italy boasts some very well-known gun manufacturers such as Beretta, making its community one that is passionate about hunting game.

Avid hunters can choose between walk-up wing shooting of fowl such as partridges and quail to a driven shoot, stalking wild boar and deer. Hunting is reserved for the picturesque Italian countryside in the Sardinia, Tuscany, and Umbria regions.

The practice is strictly regulated with permits, quotas, and designated hunting areas to ensure year-round controlled activity.

How Italian Food Took the World by Storm

Some readers will be surprised to know that almost 30 years ago, Italian food was considered food for the peasants. There were no Italian chef sensations and no fancy toppings and gelato to have for dessert.

It was still very much loved, even back then. Patrons fondly classified it as pizza with sauces. Since then, Italian food and Mediterranean food, in general, have revolutionized and emerged as gastronomic excellence. Today it is classed as one of the healthiest lifestyles to adapt, with its plethora of authentic classical dishes on offer and culture-centric lifestyles.

The 80s saw chefs making use of and working for the fresh, wholesome ingredients that have become a given in today's modern Italian kitchens. Back then, they did not have access to truffles, prosciutto, or even extra-virgin olive oil. Everything we know about Italian cooking had to be improvised in the earlier years.

Known for its cultural diversity, thanks to a wide variety of different influences over the year by various civilizations, many Italian dishes are simplistic in nature with high flavor profiles.

Italian cooking is centered around the quality of the ingredients being used in the dish instead of swanky cooking methods.

The Italian Kitchen Icon: aka Nonna!

The matriarch of any Italian *famiglia* is lady *nonna*! Who is lady nonna, you may ask? It is none other than the straight-arrow and soft-faced grandma. Unlike many other languages, in the Italian lexicon, the word nonna stays as is. There are no abbreviations and no other pet names used in the traditional sense of the word. *La nonna* is the one that you turn to when you feel like a treat; she is the stalwart and the go-to feminine role model that will pass her secret recipes on to you— well, if you ask nicely, that is.

She radiates love, care, and understanding. She is loud, and she is proud! But make no mistake! Nonna is no pushover, and as much as she loves you, she will put you back on the straight and narrow when you bend your nose out of line. *Un saluto alla vostra nonna!* (Greetings to your grandmother!)

Products of Genuine Italian Origin

Italians are proud custodians of the authenticity and quality associated with their produce. This ensures that they stand out above illicit and counterfeit products inferior in nature that are being passed off as genuine to the public.

Italy has the largest selection of these products on the entire European continent. These products are shielded for their authenticity, classic taste, and components that make them unique and that are native to their region of origin.

The region, or area of origin, refers to the geographic location (in one of Italy's 20 regions) where the product was cultivated by the environmental factors that played a role in the creation thereof, such as water, soil, climate, etc.

Other influences that lend these products their "certificate of excellence" stamp of approval are the culturally affluent history and the covert cooking methods that have made them a success.

Any consumer that invests in the DOP and IGP labeled products has chosen quality.

Unpacking the various labels of authenticity:

Indicazione Geografica Protetta (I.G.P.)

Also known as the Protected Geographical Indication (P.G.I.). This is reserved for products unique to the 20 regions. This seal provides a sense of surety to the consumer when it comes to both quality and authenticity.

Denominazione di Origine Protetta (D.O.P.)

Otherwise known as Protected Designation of Origin (P.D.O.). Similar to its I.G.P. counterpart, this seal represents genuineness and a quality product produced in one of the 20 regions of Italy. The difference between I.G.P. and D.O.P. is that with D.O.P., every detail in the production process is unique to the region of origin, from the cradle to the grave.

In the case of I.G.P., the minimum requirement is for at least one process to be unique to the area of origin.

Specialità Tradizionale Garantita (S.T.G.)

Translated in English as Traditional Specialty Guaranteed (T.S.G.). This label indicates that this particular product (authentic dish or agricultural product) has a set of original features that distinguishes it from other products in the same category.

Some of these features include being made from traditional ingredients or made using traditional cooking processes. It does not have to be mapped to a specific Italian region, as long as the other two conditions mentioned above have been met.

The Essential Pantry Staples for Italian Cooking

With this list of ingredients, you can stock your pantry with the must-have ingredients when cooking Italian food. It can also serve a dual purpose, in that this can form part of your Italian shopping list:

- oo flour
- All-purpose flour
- Almond flour
- Arborio rice
- A selection of bell peppers
- A selection of dried pasta (Spaghetti, pasta *corta*)
- Balsamic vinegar
- Basil
- Breadcrumbs
- Black peppercorns (freshly ground)
- Canned beans
- Canned tomatoes (peeled, San Marzano is the best)
- Capers
- Carrots
- Celery
- Chicken broth
- Cheeses
- Coffee
- Dried oregano
- Extra virgin olive oil
- Garlic
- Lemon juice
- Italian spices and seasoning
- Nutella or homemade *gianduja*
- Olives
- Onions

- Parmesan cheese
- Polenta
- Porcini mushrooms
- Salt-packed anchovies
- Selection of salamis, sausages, and meats
- Tomato passata (puree)
- Tomato paste
- Truffle oil
- Tuna in olive oil
- White wine vinegar

Wine (for cooking and drinking, of course)

Chapter 1:
Perfect Antipasti

Italians are pioneers when it comes to food. Not only is the food healthier, but describing a typical Italian scene, one finds animated chatter, loud conversations, and people eating slowly, savoring every last morsel on their plates.

Before delving into antipasti, there is one important factor to mention, and that is the correct pronunciation of the word. No one wants to walk around with a scarlet-lettered T for tourist!

Antipasti is deemed the starter, and you will find these typical platters on the table, served as a first course during a traditional Italian family dinner.

Customarily these jaw-droppingly colorful platters serve the purpose of setting the stage for the feast that is about to start. A primary component of these platters is the selection of different hams prevalent.

The Italian Ham Selection

Culatello: This ham originated from the Emilia-Romagna region. It is similar to prosciutto, except that this is made from the meat on the hind leg.

Pancetta: This ham is made from the same cut as bacon but is salted and air-cured instead.

Prosciutto: A dry-cured ham that is served by slicing it thinly before adding it to the platter. It can be subdivided in:

- Crudo di Cuneo, *PDO*, (Piedmont)
- Prosciutto Amatriciano, *PGI*, (Lazio)
- Prosciutto di Carpegna, *PDO*, (Marche)
- Prosciutto di Modena, *PDO*, (Emilia-Romagna)
- Prosciutto di Norcia, *PGI*, (Umbria)
- Prosciutto di Parma, *PDO*, (Emilia-Romagna)
- Prosciutto di San Daniele, *PDO*, (Friuli-Venezia Giulia)
- Prosciutto di Sauris, *PGI*, (Friuli-Venezia Giulia)
- Prosciutto Toscano, *PDO*, (Tuscany)
- Prosciutto Veneto Berico-Euganeo, *PDO*, (Veneto)

Speck: a dry-cured meat similar to that of prosciutto, as it is also made from the hind legs, but in this instance, the difference is that Speck is smoked and also has a more robust flavor in comparison to prosciutto. It has earned the label of P.G.I.

Guanciale: This meat is very fatty on the palate and is made from the cheeks of the pigs. Guanciale is dried for a period of three months to get the best out of the flavor.

Coppa: Part of the salami family and is air-cured. The meat is taken from the shoulder or the neck of the pig.

Antipasti Recipes You Can Try at Home

Taralli Le Puglia

Region of Origin: Apulia (Puglia)

Wine Pairing: Rivera Bombino Bianco

Time: 1 hour, 30 minutes

Serving Size: sufficient for 8 persons

Prep Time: 25 minutes

Cooking Time: 65 minutes

Ingredients:

- 19 oz all-purpose flour

- Extra flour for kneading
- 2 teaspoons sea salt
- 1/4 cup extra-virgin olive oil
- ⅔ cup dry white wine
- Baking sheet lined with parchment paper

Directions:

1. Add flour and sea salt to a bowl. Gradually add the oil while stirring well. Repeat the process with the white wine.

2. Transfer the dough to a lightly floured surface and knead for at least 10 minutes. Do this until you have

achieved a smooth dough with a springy consistency.

3. Preheat the oven to 374°F.

4. Cut the dough into pieces as large as an olive. Roll it in a rope, about ½ cm in thickness. Join the ends together, and firmly press together. Set aside. Repeat the process until all the dough has been rolled and formed.

5. Bring a pot of water to a boil and divide the taralli into small batches. Cook all the taralli in the water until they float to the surface.

6. Transfer them to a plate lined with kitchen towels to drain. Once they are drained, arrange them on the waiting baking sheets.

7. Bake them for 40 minutes until golden brown. Remove from the oven and allow to cool.

Parma Ham Pockets With Asparagus and Peas

Region of Origin: Emilia-Romagna

Wine Pairing: Prosecco, Malvasia, Sauvignon Blanc, Pinot Grigio, Lambrusco

Time: 25 minutes

Serving Size: 12 portions

Prep Time: 25 minutes
Ingredients:

- 2 oz asparagus
- 2 oz fresh peas, shelled
- 4.5 oz squacquerone cheese
- 4.5 oz ricotta
- 1 oz grated pecorino cheese
- 12 slices Parma ham

Directions:

1. Start by washing the asparagus in warm water. Using a potato peeler, cut 12 ribbons, and set aside.

2. Add the peas and remaining asparagus into a pot of boiling water, and blanch for five minutes. Remove from the stove and allow to cool.

3. Finely chop the blanched peas and asparagus with a sharp paring knife.

4. Add the ricotta, squacquerone, and the pecorino into a separate bowl and gently fold together until a stiff consistency has been achieved.

5. Combine the peas and the asparagus into the cheese, and mix until thoroughly combined.

6. Open the ham and place it on a flat surface—spoon 1 serving of the mixture in the middle of the ham.

7. Gather each piece of Parma ham up, and twist it into a pocket/parcel.

8. Tie the elongated top part with a piece of asparagus ribbon. Plate and serve.

Pepperoni all'Acciuga

Meaning: Pepperoni with Anchovy

Region of Origin: Piedmont

Wine Pairing: Syrah, Nero'd Avola

Time: 60 minutes

Serving Size: 6 portions

Prep Time: 10 minutes

Cooking Time: 50 minutes

Ingredients:

- 2 cups red bell peppers
- 2 cups yellow bell peppers
- 2 oz fresh parsley
- 24 anchovy fillets
- 1 garlic clove, peeled
- 2 tablespoons capers
- 2 oz stale bread - crusts removed
- 1 tablespoon white wine vinegar
- 5 oz extra-virgin olive oil
- Sea salt to taste
- Pepper to taste

Directions:

1. Preheat the oven to 392°F.

2. Poke the whole peppers with a fork multiple times, wrap in tin foil. Place them directly on the oven rack. Roast for 45 minutes, turning regularly until they are tender. Remove when done and allow to cool, still in the tinfoil.
3. Prep the salsa verde while you are waiting for the peppers, by adding the anchovies, bread, garlic, parsley, and vinegar into a food processor. Blitz continuously, adding the oil in intervals. Season to taste. Continue to blitz until a smooth and creamy consistency has been reached.
4. Remove the tinfoil from the peppers, and cut in half. Remove the seeds and the stems. Arrange the peppers on a platter, add spoonfuls of the mixture on top, and garnish them by scattering anchovy fillets on top.

Fregola Salad

Region of Origin: Sardinia

Wine Pairing: Chardonnay, Sauvignon Blanc

Time: 19 minutes

Serving Size: 4 portions

Prep Time: 10 minutes

Cooking Time: 9 minutes

Ingredients:

- 6 oz fregola

- 7 tablespoons olive oil
- 5 oz green olives, pitted and halved
- 1 garlic clove peeled and chopped finely
- 1 tablespoon marjoram
- 10 mint leaves, shredded
- 1 large fresh orange, zested
- 3 tablespoons balsamic vinegar
- Sea salt and pepper (optional)

Directions:

1. Bring salted water in a large skillet to a boil on the stove. Add the fregola to the water and cook for 9 minutes. Remove from the heat and drain the water.
2. Toss with 3 tablespoons of the olive oil. Transfer to a large, flat pan and allow to cool completely.
3. While the fregola is cooling down, add the olives, garlic, mint, marjoram, orange zest, remaining olive oil, and vinegar in a large mixing bowl. Stir to combine well.
4. Transfer the fregola to the mixture and fold it well. Season to taste and serve at room temperature.

Prosciutto Crudo & Leek Involtini

Meaning: Raw Ham & Leek Rolls

Region of Origin: Emilia-Romagna

Wine Pairing: Riesling, Moscato, Chenin Blanc, Rosé, Grenache, and Zinfandel

Time: 35 minutes

Serving Size: 4 portions

Prep Time: 10 minutes

Cooking Time: 25 minutes

Ingredients:

- 2 medium leeks
- 5 oz milk
- 2 tablespoons extra-virgin olive oil
- 2 tablespoons of flour
- 12 slices Prosciutto Crudo
- ¼ cup parmesan, grated
- ⅔ chives, chopped
- 1 tablespoon butter
- Nutmeg, sea salt, and pepper to taste

Directions:

1. Remove the outer parts of the leek. Chop the leek into 3/4 rounds. Wash with a saline solution. Drain the water on a plate lined with a kitchen towel.
2. In a large skillet, heat the olive oil. Fry the leeks until fragrant (5 minutes). The ideal is to continually stir the leeks until they have formed soft ribbons.
3. Remove the leeks from the stove, season with salt and pepper. Allow to cool in the pan.
4. Make a bechamel sauce by combining the butter and flour in a non-stick pan on low heat. Stir continuously until a paste has formed. Add the milk

and increase the heat to a medium setting. Stir until it has thickened.

5. Add a pinch of nutmeg and sea salt to taste. Continue stirring until the sauce has thickened some more. Remove from the heat, and allow to cool completely.

6. Stir the leeks and parmesan into the mixture. Prepare the prosciutto slices by adding them to a pan, leaving some space in between them.

7. Add a spoonful of the mixture onto each slice of prosciutto. Sprinkle chives on top, and roll into an involtini.

8. Once all the involtini are rolled, arrange them on plates or platters in a creative shape.

Chapter 2:
Pasta Dishes

After pizza, pasta is the next dish that embodies the essence of Italian cuisine. Pasta is the kryptonite of many people across the globe. Nearly every country in the world has taken the classic Italian dish and put their own unique spin on it.

Pasta is known as the noodles of the Italian people and is made from durum wheat. Durum wheat is low in moisture and high in gluten, making it a perfect pairing to pasta production. The grain is pressed into sheets, cut into a variety of shapes, and packaged.

Characteristics of Quality, Authentic Pasta

A quality pasta can be recognized as having the following distinguishing features:

- With the right thickness, the pasta will cook evenly in a short amount of time.
- It retains its shape, and if cooked al dente, it will remain that way and not become soggy.
- No starchy outer film will be present after it has been cooked.
- Cooking water will be clear after the pasta has been cooked. Meaning all nutrients will be retained in the pasta.
- If made from good quality gluten, the pasta will have an elastic consistency while being eaten.
- Good quality pasta is porous.

- The color will be bright yellow before and after the cooking process.

Types of Italian Pasta

There are many different types of pasta in terms of shapes. Each is unique to one of the 20 regions in Italy:

Bigoli - *Veneto*

Chitarra - *Abruzzo*

Gigli - *Tuscany*

Penne - *Campania*

Strozzapreti - *Emilia-Romagna*

Trofie - *Liguria*

Other pasta types include:

Filled pasta

Agnolotti, cappelletti, ravioli, tortellini

Long and skinny shapes

Bucatini, capellini, fusilli lunghi, linguine, spaghetti, spaghettini, vermicelli

Long ribbon-like pasta

Fettuccine, mafaldine, pappardelle, stringozzi, tagliatelle, trenette

Miniature pasta shapes

Anelli, canestrini, fregola, orzo, quadrettini, risi, stelline

Shell shaped

Conchiglie, lumache, lumaconi

Tubular

Cannelloni, ditalini, macaroni, manicotti, penne, rigatoni, paccheri, trenne, tortiglioni

Twisted

Casarecce, fusilli, gemelli, rotini, strozzapreti, trofie

Why You Should Invest in an Italian Pasta Maker

Investing in a pasta maker will elevate your Italian dishes to another level. Nothing comes close to making your own dough and then lovingly running it through the machine until perfection has been achieved.

There are a significant number of benefits when making use of a pasta machine:

- Send healthy food to your family dinner table because you are aware of the quality and nutrient value of what you made.

- Save time and get more things done in the kitchen when you have a quality pasta maker.

- Have full control over the ingredients and portions you cook and serve with.
- Discourage overeating and being overweight.
- Get the same results as an original Italian restaurant, with pasta dishes of the same quality, every time.
- Create and explore with many great pasta dishes.

Some Renowned Pasta Makers

There are many different brands of Italian Pasta Makers that can be purchased. Each brand has its own unique design, offering, and features. Some of these brands include:

1. CucinaPro Pasta Maker Deluxe
2. Imperia Pasta Maker Machine
3. Marcato Design Atlas 150 Pasta Machine
4. Norpro 1049R Pasta Machine
5. Phillips Kitchen Appliances Noodle Pasta Maker Plus
6. Weston 6 Inch Traditional Style Pasta Machine

Basic Italian Pasta Dough Recipe

Time: 1 hour, 30 minutes

Serving Size: 2 portions

Prep Time: 45 minutes

Cooking Time: 45 minutes

Ingredients:

- 1 ⅔ cups 00 flour

- 2 large eggs
- Sea salt to taste
- 1 tablespoon olive oil

Directions:

1. Clean a surface on the counter with a wet, disinfected cloth. Allow to dry.

2. Sift the flour onto the surface, make a hole in the middle. Add the remainder of the ingredients into the hole.

3. Using the fingers of one hand, gradually work in the flour until a dough has formed. Knead the dough until it has a smooth consistency (2-5 minutes). Cover the ball of dough in plastic wrap. Leave to rest for 30 minutes at room temperature.

4. Follow the instructions on the pasta maker to roll it through the machine.

Pasta Recipes for You to Try at Home

Cjalsons (Cjarsons)

Meaning: Sweet & Savoury Dumplings

Region of Origin: Friulli-Venezia Giulia

Wine Pairing: Grand Pinot Nero

Time: 1 hour, 21 minutes

Serving Size: 2 portions

Prep Time: 1 hour 15 minutes

Cooking Time: 6 minutes

Ingredients:

- ½ cup all-purpose flour
- ½ cup whole wheat flour
- 3 tablespoons butter, melted
- 1 tablespoon butter reserved
- 3 tablespoons water
- 1 egg yolk
- 2 oz minced pancetta
- ½ apple, cubed
- 1 pear, cubed
- 10 crumbled amaretti biscuits
- Sugar to taste
- Pepper to taste
- Salt to taste
- Cinnamon to taste
- Parmesan to taste

Directions:

1. In a large bowl, combine the flour, melted butter, and egg yolk. Mix well.
2. Transfer to a clean, lightly flour-dusted surface and knead until the dough becomes soft. Place in a sealable food storage bag, and refrigerate for 30 minutes.
3. Using a medium-sized frying pan, fry the pancetta on medium heat. Add the apple and pear to the pan once the pancetta changes color. Cook until the pear has just turned soft.

4. Add sugar, salt, and pepper to taste. Remove the pan from the heat, and add the crumbled amaretti to the pan. Transfer to a plate.
5. Remove dough from the fridge and roll out on a lightly floured surface until thin. A pasta machine can be used to the same effect as an alternative. Cut the dough into 3.5 mm rounds.
6. Add a teaspoon of filling to the middle of each round, brush water on the outside of the round, and fold it in half. The folded rounds should resemble a half-moon (crescent) shape. Press the edged sealing it.
7. Bring a pot of salted water to a boil on the stove. Melt the remaining butter in a separate skillet on low heat.
8. Divide the cjalsons in batches and cook them in the boiling water. Once they come to the surface, remove them from the water with a slotted spoon, and transfer them to the pan of butter.
9. Cook for 2-3 minutes, turning them gently. Sprinkle it with parmesan, pepper, and cinnamon.

Pasta alla Norma

Region of Origin: Sicily

Wine Pairing: Nero d'Avola

Time: 1 hour, 10 minutes

Serving Size: 4 portions

Prep Time: 20 minutes

Cooking Time: 50 minutes

Ingredients:

- 2 cups marinara sauce

- 2 medium eggplants, washed
- ¼ cup virgin olive oil + 1 teaspoon set aside for later
- ¼ teaspoon fine sea salt
- 8 oz spaghetti
- ½ cup fresh basil, washed and shredded
- Extra shredded basil for garnish
- 1 teaspoon chili flakes
- ½ teaspoon dried oregano
- ¾ cup parmesan cheese
- 2 large baking sheets, lined with parchment paper

Directions:

1. Preheat the oven to 425°F.
2. Wash the eggplants. Using a peeler, shave ribbons of eggplant off alternating between the skin and flesh. In the end, you will have alternating pieces of white and black ribbons.
3. Discard either end of the eggplant and cut the remainder into rounds. Place the circles on the baking sheets. Brush both sides of the rounds with olive oil. Sprinkle with fine salt.
4. Place the baking sheets in the oven and roast until golden brown on both sides. Remove from the oven and keep aside to cool.
5. Bring a pot of water to a boil, add salt and the pasta. Cook *al dente*. Drain all the water, except for ½ cup. Then return the pasta to the water.

6. In another pot, warm the marinara sauce and stir the eggplant into the sauce. Add the remainder of the olive oil, chili flakes, oregano (crush with your fingers first), and fresh basil.
7. Add the pasta and ½ pasta water to the eggplant and sauce, stir well. Add ⅔ of the cheese and keep the rest aside—season with salt and pepper to taste.
8. Transfer to bowls, garnish and serve.

Anelli alla Pecoraro

Meaning: Pecorara Rings

Region of Origin: Abruzzo
Wine Pairing: Montepulciano

Time: 75 minutes

Serving Size: 8 - 10 portions

Prep Time: 25 minutes

Cooking Time: 50 minutes

Pasta Ingredients:

- 4 cups all-purpose flour
- 1 teaspoon sea salt
- 4 extra-large eggs
- 2 tablespoons olive oil
- ¼ cup lukewarm water
- Avocado oil for frying
- 2 small eggplants cut into thin rounds
- 3 small summer squash cut into rounds

- 3 red bell peppers, finely diced
- A batch of Ragù all'Abruzzese (recipe below), heated to a simmer
- 1 cup ricotta
- Freshly grated parmesan

Ragù all'Abruzzese Ingredients:

- 5 tablespoons olive oil
- 8 oz beef, without the bone - quartered
- 6 oz pork shoulder, without the bone - cut into 3 parts
- 6 oz lamb shoulder, without the bone - cut into 3 parts
- Fine sea salt to taste
- Fresh ground pepper to taste
- 3 lbs canned tomatoes, drained
- 1 finely chopped red onion

Ragù all'Abruzzese Directions:

1. Warm the avocado oil in a large pot over medium heat. Season the meat and add to the pot. Brown on both sides for 4 minutes. Ensure that the meat is seared all over. Remove from the heat and set aside.
2. Add the tomatoes to a blender and gently blitz.
3. Return the pot to the stove and add the olive oil. Fry the onions until they become fragrant (5 minutes). Pour in the tomatoes and stir well. Bring it to a simmer.
4. Add the meat back into the pot, reduce heat to low. Cover partially with a lid and allow the sauce to simmer. Stir frequently and allow the sauce to cook for 3 hours. The meat should be tender and juicy, and the sauce should be thickened. Adjust the seasoning if desired.

5. Turn the heat off. Remove the meat from the sauce and store for later.

Pasta Directions:

1. Sift and combine the salt and flour in a food processor. Gently drizzle the olive oil in increments. Break the eggs into the mixture. Beat on a low speed.
2. Add the water in sections, and only until the dough has made miniature curds.
3. Lightly dust a work surface with additional flour and transfer the dough to the surface. Knead the dough for several minutes before wrapping it in plastic and allowing it to rest at room temperature for 30 minutes.
4. Cover the work surface with a large, clean cloth. Dust the cloth with flour. Pinch a piece of the dough, the same size as a walnut, and roll it into a rope of ⅛ inches in diameter. (Keep a bowl of water handy and wet your palms slightly to aid the rolling process.)
5. Cut the rope into 3 ½ inch lengths. Join the ends of the lengths to form a circle. Place the finished ring on the flour-dusted cloth. Continue and repeat the process until all the dough has been rolled and placed on the cloth. (If you are serving the anelli the same day, allow the rings to rest on the cloth for a few hours.)
6. Bring a large pot of salted water to a boil. Add ¼ of avocado oil to a large skillet and heat the oil on medium heat. Add the eggplant and gently fry on both sides for 4 minutes.

7. Transfer the pieces to a waiting plate lined with paper towels, and drain the oil. Fry the summer squash until golden brown and also transfer to the paper towel. Next, fry the peppers until fragrant, and also move to the plate of paper towels containing the other vegetables.
8. Move all the vegetables, with the exception of 1 cup, to the ragù. Gently stir the mixture. Once the water is boiling in the pot, work the anelli in batches to the pot.
9. Cook the anelli *al dente*. Drain all the water except for 1 cup. Return the pasta to the pot and coat with two-thirds of the sauce.
10. Dish and serve with parmesan and ricotta on top.

Bucatini all'amatriciana

Region of Origin: Lazio

Wine Pairing: Sangiovese

Time: 25 minutes

Serving Size: 8 - 10 portions
Prep Time: 5 minutes

Cooking Time: 20 minutes

Ingredients:

- 235 oz peeled Italian tomatoes (canned & drained)
- ¼ cup extra-virgin olive oil
- 1 tablespoon extra-virgin olive oil (additional)
- 1 large red onion, finely chopped

- 2 small chilies, finely chopped and stemmed
- 6 oz pancetta, thinly sliced
- 2 ½ lbs bucatini pasta
- ½ cup pecorino cheese
- 2 tablespoons additional pecorino cheese
- Fine sea salt to taste

Directions:

1. Crush the tomatoes with your hands over a large bowl. Heat the olive oil in a large frying pan. Add the onion and chilies to the pan, and cook for 5 minutes, until fragrant.
2. Next, add the pancetta and cook for 10 minutes. Add the crushed tomatoes and juiced to the pan and reduce it to low heat. Cook for 40 minutes, occasionally stirring until the sauce has thickened. Season with salt.
3. Bring the pasta to a boil in a large pot with salted water—cook the pasta *al dente*. Drain the water and return the pasta to the pot after draining it with a strainer.
4. Add the pecorino and sauce to the pasta in the pot and coat well.

Spaghetti alla Marchigiana

Region of Origin: Marche

Wine Pairing: Zinfandel

Time: 20 minutes

Serving Size: 4 servings

Prep Time: 10 minutes

Cooking Time: 10 minutes

Ingredients:

- 14 oz spaghetti

- 6 oz guanciale, cubed
- 7 oz olive oil
- 1 medium red onion, coarsely chopped
- 1 garlic clove, chopped
- 1 fresh chili pepper
- 8 oz pecorino cheese
- Seasoning to taste
- Dried oregano to taste

Directions:

1. Place the spaghetti in a large pot with salted water and cook *al dente*. In a medium skillet, fry the guanciale, onion, and chili in olive oil on low heat.
2. When the guanciale is crisped, add the onion and the garlic and continue to fry. Add seasoning to taste.
3. Remove the pan from the heat and set aside. Plate the spaghetti into bowls and sprinkle some pecorino on top. Pour the onion mixture on top, mix well and serve.
4. Finish off with some pecorino and freshly ground pepper to taste.

Agnolotti del Plin

Region of Origin: Piedmont

Wine Pairing: Ruché

Time: 2 hours

Serving Size: 6 servings

Prep Time: 20 minutes

Cooking Time: 10 minutes

Pasta Ingredients:

- 400g 00 flour
- 4 eggs

Filling Ingredients:

- 14 oz beef brisket, diced
- 1 oz all-purpose flour
- 1 medium red onion, coarsely chopped
- 2 tablespoons olive oil
- 6 oz dry red wine
- ½ cabbage, chopped roughly
- 2 oz grated Grana Padano
- Fine sea salt and ground pepper to taste

Sauce Ingredients:

- 4 oz unsalted butter
- grated Grana Padano

Directions:

1. Starting with the filling, coat the beef with flour, and shake off excess. Heat 1 oz oil in a large frying pan and brown the meat, searing it on all sides. Add the onion and wine to the pan.
2. Reduce the heat, and allow the alcohol to evaporate, cover the meat with boiling water and cook for 1 hour until tender and juicy. Adjust seasoning and remove from the heat.
3. Place a large pot on the stove and bring salted water to a boil. Add the cabbage to the water and braise for a few minutes. Drain through a strainer and allow to cool.
4. Remove the meat from the liquid and chop finely with the cooled cabbage. Add the grated cheese and season according to taste.
5. Mix until well combined, cover with cling wrap and allow to rest.
6. Moving on to the pasta dough, sift the flour on a clean, dry surface and make a hole in the middle. Crack the eggs into the hole and mix bits of flour in at a time using the fingers of one hand.
7. Knead the dough into a smooth ball with an elastic consistency. Press it flat into a disc shape. Wrap it in cling wrap and allow to rest for 30 minutes at room temperature.
8. Divide the pasta into three equal parts and roll out on a lightly floured surface or through a pasta machine. Trim into long rectangular shapes.
9. Spoon the mixture into the bottom half of each of the 3 rectangles. Fold the sheet over to cover the filling, allowing for ½ inch between. Fold the pasta

into small rectangles, sealing the edges by pressing down.

10. Bring a large pot of water to a boil, with added salt. In a medium skillet, melt the butter over mediumheat.

11. Cook the plin (pasta) in the boiling water until they float to the surface. Drain on a paper towel and transfer to the pan of melted butter. Turn frequently until they are well coated on both sides in the butter.

12. Dust with Grana Padano and serve immediately.

Chapter 3:
Meat, Poultry, and Salumi

There are various types of meat, poultry, and salumi or cured meats in Italy, and these can even be looked at granularly in detailed subcategories:

Beef

The four most popular beef producing regions in Italy are Piedmont, Umbria, Marche, Abruzzo, Molise, Emilia-Romagna, Campania, Lazio, and Tuscany.

They are responsible for breeding cattle from which the meat can yield 22 different cuts to be used in classic Italian cooking.

Bresaola

A dry-cured meat from the Lombardy region. Cut from the fillet and can be purchased aged.

Veal

Veal is cows that are less than a year old. It has a very delicate taste in comparison to other beef cuts and also lighter in color.

Poultry

Chicken

Both hens and roosters are used in Italian cooking, with the hens being more common. Chickens are classified by age:

1. Broiler (Pollastro) is 3 to 4 months old and weighs between 21 to 28 oz.
2. Pollo di Grano is 6 months old and weighs 2 lbs.
3. Roaster (Pollo/Pollastra) is about 16 weeks old and weighs between 2 to 2.5 lbs.
4. Capon (Galetto) is male and about 6 months old.
5. Gallo is a male which is two years old and is tough to eat.
6. Gallina is a female, which is old and is only suitable for its fat and making soup.

Duck

Both wild and domesticated species are used for cooking purposes. Duck meat pairs well with flavors such as tangerine, onions, prunes, cherries, olives, and red wine.

Goose

Goose is predominantly consumed during the Italian festive seasons. The meat is dark in color and goose liver is also used to create pâtés.

Pork

Guanciale

Also known as pork cheeks. It is aged for a minimum period of three months. The triangular shape is similar in texture to that of pancetta, except for the pepper-coated exterior.

Lardo

This is a type of hardened fat that is located in the neck region of the pig. It has a beautiful, delicate aroma.

Pancetta

Also commonly known as *streaky bacon* in American terms. It is made from the belly of the pig and is characterized by layers of alternating meat and fat.

Pork

Mostly used for making all the dry-cured cold cuts such as *salumi* and sausages. Both domestic as well as wild boar can be eaten.

Prosciutto

This cured meat is made from the hind legs of pigs, boars, deer, goats, buffalo, and turkey. It can be consumed *crudo* (raw) on its own or enjoyed on a platter with other cold cuts.

Salumi

It is recommended to instead invest in whole *salumi* as opposed to individual slices. Get the most out of this dish by slicing it at home and consuming it within the span of a few days.

Sausage

Sausages can be made from any of the meat that is produced in Italy. Each region has its own unique spin on the type of sausage it produces.

Lamb

Lamb is a popular choice of meat right through the year in certain regions of Italy. Mutton is a very uncommon occurrence in Italy. There are four types of lamb in this country, and they are *abbacchio* (baby lamb), *agnello* (spring lamb), *agnellone* (lamb), *pecora* (mutton).

Venison/Game

Wild boar can be wild or semi-wild, and a species known as *meticcio*, which is a culmination of breeding a domestic pig with a wild boar, is prevalent in commercial swine production.

Moreish Meat, Poultry, and Salumi Recipes

Goulash Triestino

Region of Origin: Friuli-Venezia Giulia

Time: 80 minutes

Serving Size: 6 - 10 servings

Prep Time: 20 minutes

Cooking Time: 60 minutes

Ingredients:

- ⅓ cup avocado oil
- 2 large red onions, cut into quarters
- 2 teaspoons kosher salt
- 2 lbs beef round steak cut into cubes

- 2 teaspoons smoked paprika
- 1 teaspoon oregano (dried)
- 1 twig of fresh rosemary
- 3 cups cold water
- 1 tablespoon 00 flour
- 4 tablespoons pasta di pomodoro
- Dollop of sour cream

Directions:

1. Starting with a large skillet, heat the avocado oil. Add the onions and toss in the oil, cooking until fragrant and soft on medium heat.
2. Spread out the onion evenly on the bottom of the pan. Add the cubed beef on top of the onions in one layer. Add salt, rosemary, and paprika. Cover the pan and allow the meat to stew without stirring. Check occasionally to see that the sauce and meat are not burning.
3. After half an hour, cover the pan only partially, lower the heat and stir up the onions and beef. Continue this process for another 30 minutes.
4. Combine the water and flour into the pan. Whisk until the mixture is lump-free and add the tomato paste. Frequently stir the mixture, gently folding the tomato-flour paste into the meat and onions.
5. Cook for 45 minutes to 1 hour. The meat should be tender and the sauce slightly thickened. Adjust seasoning if desired. Allow to stand for a few hours.
6. Reheat the mixture on low heat, adding a little water if required. Serve warm with a dollop of sour cream.

Smacafam

Meaning: Crush-hungry

Region of Origin: Trentino-Alto Adige

Wine Pairing: Rotari Brut

Time: 70 minutes

Serving Size: 8 servings

Prep Time: 30 minutes

Cooking Time: 40 minutes

Smacafam Ingredients:

- 2 tablespoons extra-virgin olive oil
- 1 oz lardo
- 1 red onion, thinly sliced
- 2 garlic cloves, diced
- 4 Italian pork sausages, coarsely rounded
- 6 oz portobello mushrooms, diced
- 1 cup red wine
- 7 oz canned tomatoes
- 1 sprig fresh rosemary

Polenta Ingredients:

- 3 cups chicken stock
- 6 oz polenta
- 1 oz unsalted butter, cubed
- Parmesan cheese, grated (to taste)

- 2 cups of water

Directions:

1. Combine the stock and water in a large pot to boil on medium heat. Add the polenta and stir continuously. Add seasoning and simmer, stirring frequently for 30 minutes. Stir in the butter and 1 oz of the parmesan. Turn the heat on the lowest setting to keep the polenta warm.
2. Heat the oil and the lardo in a large skillet. Stir every so often until the lardo has been rendered. Add the onion and garlic and cook until fragrant. Add the sausage, brown by stirring frequently.
3. Next, add the wine and the portobello until the liquid has been reduced to half the volume. Combine the tomato and rosemary into the mixture and simmer for 5 minutes.

Lasagna Valdostana

Region of Origin: Aosta Valley

Wine Pairing: Sangiovese

Time: 50 minutes

Serving Size: 4 servings

Prep Time: 5 minutes

Cooking Time: 45 minutes

Ingredients:

- 11 oz lasagna sheets
- 11 oz fontina cheese, cubed
- 7 oz pancetta, diced
- 5 oz parmesan cheese, finely grated
- ½ white wine
- Salted butter at room temperature
- 1 tablespoon powdered nutmeg
- 2 cups milk
- Sea salt and ground pepper to taste

Directions:

1. Preheat the oven to 356°F.
2. Combine some butter and the pancetta in a skillet. Add half of the wine and reduce the heat until half of the liquid has evaporated. Remove from the heat and set aside.
3. In another non-stick pan, add the cheese, milk, nutmeg, and salt and cook on medium heat. Stir frequently until the cheese has melted.
4. Prepare an oven dish by adding a generous layer of cooking spray along the bottom and sides. Spoon some fontina sauce at the bottom. Add a layer of lasagna.
5. Next, add tablespoons of fondue and cooked ham and spread evenly with the back of a wooden spoon. Sprinkle grated parmesan and freshly ground pepper. Repeat the process until all the ingredients have been used.
6. Bake in the oven for 30 minutes. Turn off the heat and keep the dish inside the oven for another 5 minutes. Serve and enjoy!

Saltimbocca

Meaning: Jumps in the mouth

Region of Origin: Lazio

Wine Pairing: Malbec, Cabernet Sauvignon

Time: 50 minutes

Serving Size: 4 servings

Prep Time: 5 minutes

Cooking Time: 45 minutes

Ingredients:

- 4x veal fillets, each weighing +/- 3 ounces
- 8 slices prosciutto
- 16 marjoram leaves
- 2 oz unsalted butter
- ½ cup red wine
- Fine sea salt and black pepper to taste
- Olive oil

Directions:

1. Using 2 sheets of parchment paper, place each fillet in the middle thereof. Roll each of them out to 5 mm thickness. Season with salt and pepper.
2. Add 2 marjoram leaves and 2 slices of prosciutto to the top of each fillet. Fold in the edges.

3. Heat 1 teaspoon of olive oil in a large skillet. Sauté each fillet on all sides for 2 minutes. Remove the fillets from the pan and place on a cutting board to rest for a few minutes.
4. Heat the unsalted butter in the same pan as the fillets until the butter is browned. Add the wine and whisk until emulsified.
5. Divide the fillets into 4 serving dishes and dress with the butter sauce.

Pampanella Molisana

Meaning: Spicy roast pork from Molise

Region of Origin: Molise

Wine Pairing: Sparkling Glera Prosecco

Time: 50 minutes

Serving Size: 4-6 servings

Prep Time: 5 minutes

Cooking Time: 45 minutes

Ingredients:

- 3 lbs mixed pork cuts
- Sea salt, powdered garlic, and white wine vinegar to taste
- 5 tablespoons chili flakes or powder
- 5 tablespoons sweet, unsmoked paprika

Directions:

1. Ask your butcher to make ¾ inch slices to the bone of the pork cuts. Place the meat snugly together in an oven-proof dish of 9 inches in diameter.
2. Prepare the chili and paprika rub by combining them and adjusting the spice level as desired.
3. Sprinkle the meat with sea salt and the powdered garlic. All the meat should be covered, but not overly so.
4. Repeat the same process with the chili-paprika rub. Ensure all areas, both inside and out, are covered with the rub. Marinate in the fridge for at least 3 hours or overnight.
5. Preheat the oven to 350°F. Measure a piece of parchment paper that has the circumference of covering the meat in the dish completely.
6. Wet the parchment paper slightly and wring out excess water. Cover the meat with the wet parchment paper and tuck the sides in to seal the dish. Cover the dish with tin foil and bake in the oven for 1 hour 50 minutes.
7. Remove from the oven, drizzle lightly with white wine vinegar. Cover and return to the oven for 10 minutes.

Chapter 4:
Italian Fish Cuisine

Feast of the Seven Fishes

The exact origin of this tradition is a bone of contention. It comprises a sit-down dinner table feast where a total of seven fish dishes are consumed.

Tradition dictates that it has to be seven different types of fish, prepared seven different ways.

It appears that this culinary observance is more popular amongst Americans, and very few Italians have adopted this part of their heritage. This practice is typically done every Christmas Eve. The number seven is believed to be connected to numerous Catholic symbols.

In the bible, the number seven is repeated more than 700 times. According to the Roman Catholic Church, the seven courses of the feast are linked to the seven days of Creation and the seven deadly sins as shown in (*The Origin of the Feast of the Seven Fishes*, 2019)

If you are a family of pescatarian food lovers and you would like to try your hand at this feast, I can recommend the following dishes for you to try (in sequential order):

1. *Acciughe Marinate alla Ligure (Marinated Anchovies)*
2. *Brodetto di Branzino (Wild Sea Bass Soup)*
3. *Crudo di Pesce (Fish Tartare)*

4. *Paccheri con Sugo di Mare (Seafood Pasta)*
5. *Pesce al Forno (Baked Fish)*
6. *Pesce alla Griglia (Grilled Fish)*
7. *Pesce in Umido (Fish with Roasted Fennel and Taggiasca Olives)*

Fregola allo Scoglio

Region of Origin: Sardinia

Wine Pairing: Combinate Vermentino

Time: 45 minutes

Serving Size: 4 servings

Prep Time: 20 minutes

Cooking Time: 25 minutes

Ingredients:

- 1 teaspoon saffron
- ¼ dry white wine
- 2 tablespoons extra-virgin olive oil
- ½ lb shrimp, deveined and shelled
- ½ lb scallops
- 1 small red onion, finely chopped
- 2 minced garlic cloves
- 2 cups chicken stock
- 1 cup fregola
- ½ clams, scrubbed
- 2 tablespoons freshly minced parsley
- Sea salt and freshly ground pepper to taste

Directions:

1. In a pestle and mortar, crush the saffron, add the wine, and put aside for later.
2. Add the olive oil to a large, cast-iron pot and heat over high heat. Add the shrimp and sear for 1 minute on each side. Place the seared shrimp in a separate bowl. Add the scallops and repeat the process. Move to the same bowl containing the shrimp.
3. Pour the remaining oil, garlic, and onion into the pot. Cook until fragrant. Reduce to medium heat and season with salt and pepper as desired.
4. Combine the clams into the pot, and cover with the lid—steam for 3 minutes. Add the shrimp and scallops to the pot. Cook for 3 more minutes.
5. Spoon the mixture into 4 waiting bowls, sprinkle with parsley and serve.

Brodetto alla Vastese

Meaning: Spicy roast pork from Molise

Region of Origin: Abruzzo

Wine Pairing: Trebbiano d'Abruzzo

Time: 1 hour, 20 minutes

Serving Size: 4 servings

Prep Time: 20 minutes

Cooking Time: 1 hour

Ingredients:

- 3.5 lbs fish
- 4 cloves garlic
- A few slices of bread
- 8 cuttlefish
- ½ cup extra-virgin olive oil
- ¼ cup of red onion
- Fine sea salt to taste
- 8 medium-sized shrimp (deveined and shelled)
- 2 cups tomato purée
- 1 tablespoon fresh parsley
- 1 large chili pepper
- 1 oz muscles
- 1 oz clams

Directions:

1. Heat the olive oil in a large skillet over medium heat. Combine the tomato and garlic and cook until fragrant. Add the tomato and parsley. Bring to a boil for 5 minutes.
2. Pour 2 cups of boiling water into the skillet, add the cuttlefish and boil for 10 minutes.
3. Add the other seafood to the pan at a gradual pace. Continue cooking for another 10 minutes. If the juices are too thick, then dilute with some warm water.
4. Fry the slices of bread in a pan with some olive oil until crisp. Dip the bread into the seafood dish and sauce.

Risotto alla Pescatora

Region of Origin: Campania

Drink Pairing: Bicchiere di vino bianco

Time: 46 minutes

Serving Size: 4 servings

Prep Time: 20 minutes

Cooking Time: 26 minutes

Ingredients:

- 14 oz Arborio rice
- 1.1 lb mixed seafood
- 3 oz olive oil
- 1 garlic clove
- 1 medium-sized mild chili
- 2 tablespoons tomato paste
- 3 ½ oz white wine
- 4 cups fish stock
- ½ teaspoon fresh black pepper
- Sea salt to taste
- Parsley to taste

Directions:

1. If you are using frozen fish, defrost, open the packet and dry with kitchen towels.
2. Heat the olive oil in a large pan over low heat. Add the garlic, onion, and the chili and cook until fragrant.

3. As soon as the garlic is golden, remove it from the pan and discard it. Remove the chili from the pan and discard it.
4. Turn the heat to medium and add the seafood to the pan. Combine well with the oil, and cook for just 3 minutes.
5. Remove the seafood with a slotted spoon and place it aside in a bowl. Cover the bowl with tinfoil.
6. Add the rice to the pan and coat well. Stir for 2 minutes. Add the wine and keep stirring until it evaporates.
7. Add the stock in spoonfuls to the pan and reduce to low heat. During this process, keep stirring gently at a continuous pace.
8. When half of the stock is added, pour in the tomato paste. Stir until an orange-colored sauce is achieved. Adjust the salt and pepper seasoning if required.
9. Add the seafood to the pan, stirring frequently until the rice is *al dente*. Add the parsley and stir.

Lumache alla Bresciana

Region of Origin: Lombardy

Drink Pairing: Montonale La Venga

Time: 3 hours

Serving Size: 4 servings

Prep Time: 2 hours

Cooking Time: 60 minutes

Ingredients:

- 7 oz snail/escargot meat
- 1 finely chopped red onion
- 1 tablespoon tomato paste
- 14 oz roughly shredded spinach
- ¼ cup olive oil
- ⅔ oz salted butter
- 1 tablespoon dried parsley
- ⅔ grated parmesan
- 1 carrot, peeled and rounded
- 2 cloves garlic
- 2 spring onions, finely chopped
- 1 medium celery stalk coarsely rounded
- Fine sea salt and pepper to taste

Directions:

1. Bring a large pot of salted water to a boil. Add the snail meat. Simmer for 10 minutes and scoop off any residue that might rise to the surface. Remove from the pot with a slotted spoon, shaking off excess water.
2. Place the meat in a bowl and cover with white wine vinegar. Marinade for 3 hours. Rinse under running water and set aside.
3. Add the carrot, spring onion, and celery to a pan of cold water together with the snail meat and white wine.
4. Bring the liquid to a boil, and simmer for 1 hour. Separate the meat from the rest of the pan, place in a bowl, and cover with a clean dishcloth.

5. In a large saucepan, melt the butter and oil together. Place all of the spinach in the pot. Add the onion and garlic and cook until fragrant.
6. Add the meat and cook for another 3 minutes. Next, add the tomato paste and stir well.
7. Combine the spinach with the rest of the ingredients in the pot. Cook covered for 20 minutes on low heat. Adjust seasoning if required.
8. Stir in the parsley and cook for 20 minutes.

Bagna cauda

Meaning: *hot bath*
Region of Origin: Piedmont

Wine Pairing: Nebbiolo

Time: 20 minutes

Serving Size: 6 servings

Prep Time: 5 minutes

Cooking Time: 15 minutes

Ingredients:

- ¾ cup extra-virgin olive oil
- 6 tablespoons salted butter at room temperature
- 12 fillets of anchovy
- Mixed choice vegetables cut into small cubes
- 1 lb Italian bread, cut into sections of 2 inches

Directions:

1. Combine the butter, anchovies, and oil into a food processor and blend well. Transfer the mixture to a medium-sized skillet.
2. Cook on a low heat for 15 minutes, stirring on occasion. Season with salt and pepper.
3. Transfer mixture to a fondue pot over heat. Serve with bread and fresh vegetables.

Whitebait With Dill Mayonnaise

Region of Origin: Liguria

Wine Pairing: Muscadet, Picpoul

Time: 30 minutes

Serving Size: 1 serving

Prep Time: 10 minutes

Cooking Time: 20 minutes

Ingredients:

- 2 tablespoons cumin seeds
- 2 tablespoons mayonnaise
- 1 cup extra-virgin olive oil
- 2 oz 00 flour
- 16 oz whitebait
- 1 lime
- Fresh dill chopped
- Fish spice, sea salt, and freshly ground pepper to taste

Directions:

1. Heat the olive oil in a large skillet over a medium heat.
2. In a large mixing bowl, sift the flour. Crush the cumin seeds and add this to the sifted flour. Season to taste with the spices.
3. Portion the whitebait in batches. Coat in the flour and fry in the oil until crispy and golden brown. Remove from the pan and drain on a plate with kitchen towels.
4. Combine the dill and the mayonnaise and add freshly squeezed lime to taste. Put the mayo dip in the middle of a platter, add the whitebait and serve.

Chapter 5:
Rice Dishes for the Win

Italy is a rice-producing country that yields approximately 1.3 million tons of rice annually. The majority of this product is then shipped out to its neighboring countries on the European continent.

Rice production predominately comes from the Lombard, Piedmont, and Veneto regions. These regions have been grain producers since the 15th century.

The Italians boast modern and sustainable techniques that are aimed at preserving the country's resources.

Rice Is Born in Water and Must Die in Wine

Risotto ai Mirtilli e Speck

Region of Origin: Trentino-Alto Adige

Wine Pairing: Dogajolo Bianco

Time: 20 minutes

Serving Size: 1 serving

Prep Time: 5 minutes

Cooking Time: 15 minutes

Ingredients:

- 13 oz carnaroli rice
- 7 oz blueberries
- 3.5 oz speck, cut into strips
- 4 cups vegetable stock
- 1 oz unsalted butter
- 1 oz grated parmesan cheese
- 1 small red onion
- Fresh rosemary
- ½ glass of red wine
- Olive oil
- Salt and pepper to taste

Directions:

1. Heat a knob of butter and the blueberries in a large skillet. Fry for a few minutes, and then cover with a lid and cook until soft. Transfer to a blender and combine on high speed until a purée-like consistency has been achieved. Put the purée aside for now.
2. In another pan, heat a few teaspoons of oil. Chop the onion, cook until fragrant and then brown the speck. Stir the mixture occasionally.
3. Add the rice and toast it for 3 minutes. Increase the heat to a high setting. Add the red wine and allow the liquid to evaporate. Lower the heat and add ladles full of stock at a time while the risotto is cooking.
4. When the risotto is halfway done, add the blueberry purée to the pan. Stir frequently. If more moisture is needed, keep adding spoons full of the stock.
5. When the risotto is done, remove the pan from the heat, add the grated cheese, rosemary, and remaining butter. Stir well.
6. Let the mixture rest for a few minutes. Serve topped with blueberries.

Italian Wild Rice Soup

Region of Origin: Emilia-Romagna

Time: 8 hours, 25 minutes

Serving Size: 8 servings

Prep Time: 25 minutes

Cooking Time: 8 hours

Ingredients:

- 1 lb pork meat
- 4 cups of warm water
- Extra-virgin olive oil
- 3.5 oz beef broth or stock
- 1 can diced tomatoes
- 6 oz tomato paste
- 1 large red onion, chopped
- ¾ cup uncooked wild rice, drained and rinsed
- 6 cloves minced garlic
- 2 tablespoons mixed herbs
- ½ teaspoon smoked paprika
- 1 teaspoon cumin seeds
- ¼ crushed chili flakes
- 19 oz shredded baby spinach
- ½ cup grated parmesan cheese
- Sea salt, pepper to taste

Directions:

1. Heat some olive oil in a large pan and add the pork. Cook until the color is no longer pink and break up the chunks of meat with a spoon. Sear on all sides.
2. Add the seared pork, water, broth, tomatoes, tomato paste, rice, garlic, mixed herbs, paprika, cumin, and seasoning to a slow cooker.
3. Cook on a low setting for 7 hours or on a high heat setting for 4 hours. Stir the spinach into the soup until well combined. Serve with grated parmesan on top.

Piedmontese Carnaroli Risotto With Veal Tongue, Hazelnuts, and Grana Padano

Region of Origin: Piedmont

Time: 70 minutes

Serving Size: 8 servings

Prep Time: 10 minutes

Cooking Time: 60 minutes

Veal Tongue Ingredients:

- 1 tongue of veal
- 1 chopped carrot (peeled)
- 1 chopped celery stalk
- 1 finely chopped red onion
- 1 bay leaf
- 2 whole black peppercorns

- 1 oz Piedmontese hazelnuts

Risotto Ingredients:

- 6.5 cups vegetable broth
- 8 oz carnaroli rice
- 2 oz unsalted butter
- 3 oz grated Grana Padano
- Olive oil
- Fine sea salt
- Freshly ground black pepper

Directions:

1. Preheat the oven to 356°F.
2. Add the tongue and all the ingredients to prepare it in a large pot. Cover everything with water and bring to a boil. Reduce the heat and cook on a simmer for 2 hours. Remove from the heat and allow to cool in the liquid.
3. After the veal has rested for 3 hours, strain through a sieve into another pan. Reduce on the stove to low heat, until the liquid is a dark, rich color.
4. Remove the tongue from the liquid, and peel with a paring knife. Place in the fridge to rest for 45 minutes.
5. Place the nuts in a food processor and grind into a powder, set aside for later.
6. Next up is the risotto. Using a large skillet, pour the stock into the pan, and heat over a medium setting.
7. Add a dash of olive oil and toast the rice for 2 minutes, stirring frequently.
8. Season the risotto to taste. Add the stock, spoonfuls at a time. Before adding the next spoonful, allow

the risotto to absorb the last round of liquid first. Stir continuously for 20 minutes, until the risotto is creamy.

9. Cut a 7 oz portion of veal into cubes. Season to taste with salt and pepper and brown in a small frying pan with a bit of olive oil.

10. As soon as the risotto is cooked, remove the pan from the heat and stir in the cheese.

Risotto Primavera

Region of Origin: Veneto

Time: 25 minutes

Serving Size: 6-8 servings

Prep Time: 15 minutes

Cooking Time: 10 minutes

Ingredients:

- 1 medium-sized carrot, peeled

- 4 tablespoons extra-virgin olive oil
- 8 ounces asparagus spears
- 1 medium zucchini seeded and trimmed
- 1 medium-sized summer squash quartered
- 4 ½ cups chicken stock
- 1 finely chopped red onion (large)
- 1 ¾ cup Arborio rice
- ¾ cup dry white wine

- 4 medium-sized carrots - peeled
- 4 oz grated parmesan
- 1 cup peas
- ¼ cup of salted butter
- ½ cup basil leaves
- ¼ cup cashew nuts
- Additional grated parmesan

Directions:

1. Cut the medium-sized carrot into strips. Heat 1 tablespoon of olive oil over medium-high heat. Add the asparagus spears, zucchini, and summer squash. Sprinkle it with salt and pepper.
2. Bring the stock to a simmer in a medium skillet over low heat. Cover and keep warm as far as possible.
3. Heat 3 tablespoons of olive oil in a large pot over medium heat. Add the onion and the 4 carrots and cook until fragrant. Add the rice and cook *al dente*. Add the wine and cook for 3 minutes. Add 1 cup of stock and carrots, simmer for 4 minutes and add 2 more cups. Cook for 10 minutes.
4. Combine the fried vegetables and 1 cup of stock. Simmer for 5 minutes.
5. Add 1 1/3 cups of the cheese, peas, butter, and another 1/2 cup broth. Simmer the mixture until the butter has melted and the rice, and veggies are tender. The risotto should be creamy. Add the basil and season with salt and pepper.

Chapter 6:
Vegetarian Dishes

One of the key characteristics of Italian cooking is the approach of having only a few fresh ingredients on hand to concoct dishes that are packed with flavor.

Some of the key vegetables that are prevalent in classic Italian cooking are (but not limited to):

- Artichokes
- Asparagus
- Aubergine
- Beans
- Beetroot
- Bell peppers
- Broccoli
- Carrots
- Cauliflower
- Celery
- Corn
- Fennel
- Greens
- Mushrooms
- Onions
- Peas
- Potatoes
- Summer squash
- Tomatoes
- Winter squash

Wholesome Vegetarian Recipes

Fave e Cicoria

Meaning: Fava bean purée with wild chicory

Region of Origin: Puglia

Time: 65 minutes

Serving Size: 4 servings

Prep Time: 5 minutes

Cooking Time: 60 minutes

Ingredients:

- 7 oz fava beans, split
- 1 bay leaf
- 1 clove garlic, crushed
- Vegetable broth
- 3.5 oz chicory
- Avocado oil
- Salt and pepper to taste

Directions:

1. In a large skillet, combine the beans, bay leaf, garlic clove, and salt. Cover with vegetable broth.
2. Simmer for 60 minutes until the beans are slushy (add more stock in spoonfuls at a time to avoid burning).

3. When a purée has formed, remove the bay leaf and the garlic clove from the mixture. Season according to taste. Add a dash of olive oil.
4. Wither the greens in a little olive oil in another skillet with a pinch of salt and a tablespoon of water.
5. Plate the purée with a dollop of wilted greens.

Erbazzone

Meaning: Swiss-chard pie

Region of Origin: Emilia-Romagna

Time: 70 minutes

Serving Size: 4 servings

Prep Time: 10 minutes

Cooking Time: 60 minutes

Dough Ingredients:

- 2 cups all-purpose flour

- Fine sea salt to taste
- Good quality olive oil
- Water

Filling Ingredients:

- 2.2 lbs swiss-chard, washed and shredded
- 3.5 oz pancetta or prosciutto

- 3 tablespoons avocado oil
- 1 red onion, coarsely diced
- 3.5 oz grated parmesan
- Salt and pepper to taste

Directions:

1. Sift the flour and salt in a large mixing bowl. Add the oil and ¾ of water. Knead into an elastic ball of dough. Place the dough in a resealable bag and refrigerate for 1 hour.
2. Chop the beetroot and blanch the stems in hot water. Drain of moisture and put aside. Heat some olive oil in a large pan on medium heat. Add the pancetta or prosciutto and cook until the fat has been rendered. Stir in the onion and cook until fragrant.
3. Combine the spinach, beet leaves, and stems. Toss in the fat. Cover the pan and allow it to cook. When the greens have withered, remove the lid and cook until the liquid has dissipated. Remove from the heat and allow to cool.
4. Preheat the oven to 392°F. Line the baking sheet with parchment paper.
5. Divide the dough into 2 equal parts. Roll out the first half as thin as possible to cover the surface of the baking sheet. Arrange on the lined baking sheet.
6. Fold the cheese into the spinach and spread the filling evenly on top of the dough. Repeat the same process with the second ball of dough and arrange this on top of the filling.
7. Fold and seal the dough's edges and brush with egg wash or a little bit of oil.
8. Bake for 30 minutes or until golden brown and crisp.

Frittata Rafano e Pecorino

Meaning: Horseradish and pecorino dish

Region of Origin: Basilicata

Time: 45 minutes

Serving Size: 6 servings

Prep Time: 10 minutes

Cooking Time: 35 minutes

Ingredients:

- 11 oz mashed spunta potatoes

- 8 free-range chicken eggs
- 3 oz grated pecorino cheese
- 1 oz horseradish
- Extra-virgin olive oil
- Sea salt and pepper to taste

Directions:

1. Preheat the oven grill section to 392°F.
2. The mash needs to be cooled down, but still warm enough, and not cook the eggs.
3. In a large skillet, heat some olive oil on medium heat. Crack the eggs into the pan and add the mashed potato. Next, add the pecorino and horseradish, seasoning to taste.

4. Cook together for 5 minutes until it becomes fragrant. Remove the pan and place it under the grill for a few minutes.

Parmigiana Stacks

Meaning: Eggplant stacks

Wine Pairing: Casascarpa

Time: 15 minutes

Serving Size: 4 servings

Prep Time: 5 minutes

Cooking Time: 10 minutes

Ingredients:

- ½ batch of marinara sauce
- 13 oz ricotta cheese
- 1 free-range chicken egg
- Garlic powder, salt, pepper to taste
- 1 cup fresh oregano
- ¼ cup grated parmesan
- 1 large eggplant
- 2 tablespoons of olive oil
- Mozzarella cheese

Directions:

1. Preheat the oven to 375°F. Prepare a large baking sheet with parchment paper.

2. Slice the eggplant into an equal number of rounds with a thickness of 1 inch each. Rub both sides (including the edges) with oil and spices. Place the rounds on the baking sheet.
3. Bake on both sides for 15 minutes, until just tender but golden in color. Remove from the oven and remove from the sheet.
4. Line the baking sheet with a fresh layer of parchment paper. Place the 4 largest rounds down first. Spread a layer of ricotta and a generous slice of mozzarella on each. Add a tablespoon of marinara sauce to each portion of eggplant. Continue the process creating 4 stacks. Save some marinara sauce for serving.
5. Return to the oven and bake for 10 minutes. Serve with marinara sauce and sprinkle parmesan on top.

Chapter 7:
Italian Bread

Italian bread is soft and light, fluffy on the inside and crisp on the outside. There are 17 types of bread that are popular amongst its patrons:

1. Tartalli
2. Piadina
3. Penia
4. Panettone
5. Pane di Altamura *DOP*
6. Pane Casareccio di Genzano *IGP*
7. Pane Carasau
8. Pandoro
9. Grissini
10. Fragguno
11. Focaccia
12. Farro della Garfagnana *IGP*
13. Faranita
14. Coppia Ferrarese *IGP*
15. Colomba Pasquale
16. Ciabatta
17. Cecìna

Italian Bread Recipes

Ligurian Focaccia

Time: 65 minutes

Serving Size: 1 flatbread

Prep Time: 5 minutes

Cooking Time: 60 minutes

Dough Ingredients:

- 1 ½ cups of tepid water
- ½ teaspoon active dry yeast
- 2 ½ teaspoons honey
- 5 ⅓ cups 00 flour
- 1 tablespoon of sea salt
- Olive oil
- Rosemary twigs
- Flaked sea salt

Brine Ingredients:

- 1 ½ teaspoons fine sea salt
- ⅓ cup tepid water

Directions:

1. Combine the water, honey, and yeast in a mixing bowl and stir until dissolved. Sift the flour and salt into a large mixing bowl and add the yeast mixture and oil. Cover and rest at room temperature for 12 hours. It needs to grow double in size.
2. Add 3 tablespoons of olive oil to a baking sheet and coat well by turning until the whole surface is covered. Pour the dough out into the baking sheet. Pour 2 tablespoons of oil on top of the dough and spread throughout.
3. Stretch the dough for 30 minutes until the bottom is completely covered and spread evenly. Press

dimples in the dough with your first 3 fingers at an angle, repeat a few times.

4. Make the brine by stirring the ingredients thereof together until the salt is dissolved. Pour over the dimples until covered. Leave to rise for 45 minutes. Preheat the oven to 450°F.

5. Sprinkle the focaccia dough with the flaky sea salt and arrange the rosemary stalks. Bake for 30 minutes. Then turn the oven to grill and crisp for 7 minutes.

6. Remove from the oven and brush with olive oil. Allow to rest for 5 minutes. Remove from the pan and serve.

Gnocchi di Pane Raffermo

Meaning: Italian Bread Dumplings

Time: 25 minutes

Serving Size: 4 servings

Prep Time: 20 minutes

Cooking Time: 5 minutes

Gnocchi Ingredients:

- 6.5 oz stale white bread
- 5 oz sultanas or raisins
- 5 oz grated parmesan
- 1 cup 00 flour
- 2 free-range chicken eggs
- 1 teaspoon ground cinnamon

- Nutmeg, sea salt to taste
- Milk

Dressing Ingredients:

- 2 oz salted butter, melted
- 2 marjoram leaves

Directions:

1. Combine the bread and milk in a large bowl and allow to rest for 15 minutes. The bread needs to be soft.
2. Soak the raisins in a separate bowl with tepid water for 5 minutes. Squash the bread with your hands, removing any excess milk.
3. In a large mixing bowl, add the bread, parmesan, nutmeg, salt, raisins, eggs, and flour. Mix with a spoon until well combined.
4. Using a large pot with plenty of salt, bring it to a boil. Add tablespoons of the mixture to the water. When the dumplings start to float on the top, remove them with a spoon, and transfer to a warm plate.
5. Warm the butter and marjoram leaves in a pan. Pour the dressing over the dumplings and sprinkle parmesan on top.

Homemade Veneto Ciabatta Bread

Time: 1 hour, 55 minutes

Serving Size: 1 loaf

Prep Time: 10 minutes

Rising Time: 1 hour, 30 minutes

Cooking Time: 25 minutes

Ingredients:

- 1 cup and 1 tablespoon of water, divided
- ½ teaspoon honey
- 2 teaspoons active dry yeast
- 2 cups and 3 tablespoons of 00 flour, divided
- 1 teaspoon fine sea salt

Directions:

1. Combine ¼ cup water, honey, and yeast in a bowl and allow to rest for 5 minutes before stirring. Sift the flour in a large mixing bowl. Make a hole in the center, and add the yeast mixture and water in the well. Mix well and when almost done, add the salt. Sprinkle the top of the dough with 1 ½ tablespoon of flour.
2. Cover the bowl with a tea towel and allow to rest for 1 hour 30 minutes.
3. Preheat the oven to 425°F. Prepare a baking sheet by lining it with parchment paper. Transfer the dough ball to the baking sheet, careful to keep the flour on top intact.

4. Using a spoon, form the dough into a log shape. In the bottom tray of the oven, place a tray with 6 ice cubes in the middle. Bake the dough for 25 minutes.

Crescia Sfogliata

Meaning: Flaky flatbread

Region of Origin: Le-Marche

Time: 45 minutes

Serving Size: 1 loaf

Prep Time: 20 minutes

Cooking Time: 25 minutes

Ingredients:

- 18 oz all-purpose flour
- 1 free-range egg
- 3 oz lard + additional 2 oz for layers
- 3 oz lukewarm milk
- 4 oz water
- 1 heaped teaspoon fine sea salt
- Freshly ground black pepper to taste

Directions:

1. Sift the flour in salt into a large mixing bowl. Add the milk, egg, and water. Mix to form a dough. Allow the dough to sit uncovered for 20 minutes. Place dough on a lightly floured surface.

2. Pull on one side of the dough and fold it into the middle. Repeat the process with the opposite side.
3. Turn the dough 90 degrees and repeat the previous step. Roll the dough over and leave to rest for 20 minutes.
4. Divide the dough into portions of 5 oz each. Pull one side of each portion to the middle section. Pull the opposite side and join them in the middle.
5. Turn the dough 90 degrees and repeat the previous step. Roll the dough over and leave to rest for 20 minutes.
6. Using a spray bottle, lightly spritz the surface with olive oil. Roll out each portion to a thickness of 2 mm.
7. Brush the flat tops with lard, dividing it into equal parts. Roll each portion up to form a tube.
8. Roll the ends inwards to each other. Heat a pancake pan to a medium heat and add a bit of olive oil.
9. Respray the working surface again with more oil and roll the dough out to a 3mm thickness.
10. Fry each flatbread for 2 minutes a side.
11. Place one crescia on a plate, add your choice of toppings. Place another crescia on top and cut into slices to serve.

Tuscan Panzanella Salad

Region of Origin: Tuscany

Time: 35 minutes

Serving Size: 6 servings

Prep Time: 10 minutes
Cooking Time: 25 minutes

Ingredients:

- 2 ½ lbs tomatoes, cubed
- 2 teaspoons fine sea salt + additional for later
- ¾ sourdough bread, cut into cubes of 1 ½ inches in diameter
- 10 tablespoons olive oil, divided
- 2 tablespoons of diced red onion
- 2 teaspoons crushed garlic
- ½ teaspoon hot mustard
- 2 tablespoons white wine vinegar
- Black pepper to taste
- ½ oz fresh basil leaves

Directions:

1. Place the tomatoes in a strainer over the sink and season with 2 teaspoons sea salt. Shake to coat well. Drain for a total of 15 minutes, tossing regularly.
2. Preheat the oven to 350°F. Combine the bread and 2 tablespoons of oil in a large mixing bowl. Shake the bread to coat it in the oil.
   Apply a generous layer of cooking spray to a large cookie sheet.
3. Move the bread to the baking sheet and bake in the oven for 15 minutes. Remove and allow to cool. Add the tomatoes, garlic, onion, mustard, and vinegar to a mixing bowl. Whisk well. Add the remainder of the olive oil to the mixture. Adjust seasoning as desired.
4. Add the toasted bread and basil to the mixture. Shake gently to coat. Allow the mixture to rest for half an hour before serving.

Chapter 8: Desserts

This is the chapter that most people probably looked forward to. There are many different dessert and pastry recipes; it was almost impossible to add just a few favorites for you to make and enjoy at home!

Delicious Italian Desserts

Pressnitz

Meaning: *"Walnut crescents"*

Region of Origin: Friuli-Venezia Giulia

Time: 60 minutes

Serving Size: 6 servings

Prep Time: 20 minutes

Cooking Time: 40 minutes

Ingredients:

- 2.5 oz sultanas
- 2.5 oz raisins
- ½ cup rum
- 5 oz walnuts
- 5 oz almonds
- 1 oz pine nuts
- 3.5 oz dark chocolate
- 3.5 oz breadcrumbs

- 5 oz granulated sugar
- ½ teaspoon cinnamon
- 3 oz candied peel
- 1 lemon zest, grated
- 1 orange zest, grated
- 2 free-range eggs
- 3 oz salted butter, melted
- 10 oz puff pastry
- Egg wash made from 1 egg yolk

Directions:

1. Soak the raisins and sultanas in the rum for 1 hour. Drain the liquid and set aside. Store the raisins and sultans for later.
2. Preheat the oven to 356°F. Combine the nuts and chocolate in a food processor, gently blitz together.
3. Pour the nuts and chocolate into a large mixing bowl. Add the raisins, sultanas, breadcrumbs, sugar, cinnamon, zests, candied peel, and stir well.
4. Beat the eggs with a fork in a small mixing bowl and add them to the mixture. Next, add a bit of rum and the melted butter. Gently stir until a paste has formed.
5. Roll out the pastry into a rectangle of 50x20 cm. Trim the edges, so they are of equal size.
6. Spoon the mixture on one side of the dough and roll up to form a sausage. Brush a little egg yolk on the edge to make it stick to the dough. Close the ends by folding the pastry under, creating a spiral-like shape.
7. Brush with egg yolk and bake for 40 minutes.

Cannoli Siciliani

Region of Origin: Sicily

Time: 1 hour, 50 minutes

Serving Size: 24 portions

Prep Time: 1 hour, 30 minutes

Cooking Time: 20 minutes

Cannoli shell ingredients:

- 2 cups 00 flour
- 1 free-range egg
- 1 tablespoon olive oil
- 1 tablespoon brown sugar
- ¼ cup red wine
- 3 tablespoons full fat milk
- 1 egg white, separated
- Olive oil for frying

Ricotta filling ingredients:

- 4 cups of ricotta
- ¾ cup icing sugar
- Pinch of cinnamon
- ½ cup of dark chocolate chips
- 1 cup finely chopped pistachios
- Additional powdered sugar for dusting on top.

Directions for the shells:

- Sift the flour in a large bowl, and make a depression in the middle. Pour in the egg, wine, sugar, and milk. Gently stir the ingredients in the middle, combining bits of flour each time. Knead into a dough ball.
- Divide the dough ball into a few equal portions. Roll them out on a lightly floured surface to ⅛ mm thickness. Cover with a clean, dry kitchen towel.
- Cut rounds of 4 inches in diameter. Repeat with all the dough. Wrap the dough pieces around a bamboo dowel or a cannoli mold. Seal the edges with the beaten egg white.
- Add the oil to a large pot, filling it halfway and then heating it. Fry the cannoli shells until golden brown. Remove from the oil and allow to drain on a plate with kitchen towel.

Directions for the filling:

1. Combine all of the ingredients in a mixing bowl until smooth. Transfer to a piping bag and pipe the mixture into the shells, equally dividing it.
2. Dip the ends of the cannoli in pistachio and chocolate chips. Dust with icing sugar.

Torta con le Mele

Meaning: Apple cake

Region of Origin: Trentino-Alto Adige

Time: 1 hour, 50 minutes

Serving Size: 24 portions

Prep Time: 1 hour, 30 minutes

Cooking Time: 20 minutes

Ingredients:

- 1 cup unsalted butter at room temperature.
- 1 ½ cup all-purpose flour, plus additional for dusting
- 1 tablespoon baking powder
- 1 teaspoon fine sea salt
- ¾ cup brown sugar
- 3 eggs
- ¼ Grappa
- 3 green apples, peeled and cored (1 apple to be thinly sliced, 2 apples coarsely chopped)

Directions for the filling:

1. Preheat the oven 350°F. Grease an 8-inch springform tin with the butter and dust lightly with flour. Shake off excess flour.
2. Sift the flour, salt, and baking powder into a medium mixing bowl. Using an electric mixer, beat

the sugar and butter until creamy. Add the eggs and Grappa, beat again.

3. Pour into the flour mixture and combine well. Stir in the 2 chopped apples.

4. Pour the mixture into the springform tin. Sprinkle the remaining apple on top. Bake for 40 minutes. Remove from the oven, and place on a cooling rack for another 15 minutes.

5. Remove from the tin, place on a platter. Dust with icing sugar, cinnamon and serve with cream, ice cream, or evaporated milk.

Pasticioto

Region of Origin: Puglia

Time: 56 minutes

Serving Size: 12 pastries

Prep Time: 30 minutes

Cooking Time: 26 minutes

Dough Ingredients:

- 1 3/4 cups all-purpose flour
- Dash of sea salt
- ½ cup brown sugar
- 1 teaspoon baking powder
- 1 free-range egg at room temperature
- 1 free-range egg yolk at room temperature
- ½ cup salted butter at room temperature + 2 tablespoons extra for later

Custard Ingredients:

- ¾ cup full fat milk
- ¾ heavy whipping cream
- 4 egg yolks
- ½ cup brown sugar
- ½ teaspoon vanilla essence
- 2 ½ tablespoons all-purpose flour
- 2 medium lemon peels

Directions for the custard:

1. Heat the milk, lemon peels, and cream over a low heat in a medium pot. Remove from the heat and allow to cool.
2. Combine the yolks and sugar in another medium-sized pot. Add the vanilla and the flour and whisk well. Remove from the heat and strain the liquid, discarding the lemon peel. Whisk until the custard is thick and lump-free. Move to a bowl and cover with cling wrap; refrigerate for 1 hour.

Directions for the dough:

1. Sift all the dry ingredients into a large mixing bowl. Combine the rest of the ingredients into another mixing bowl and beat well.
2. Make a well in the middle of the dry ingredients and combine bits of flour at a time. Once the dough has formed, roll out on a lightly floured surface until soft.
3. Wrap the dough in cling wrap and refrigerate for half an hour. Preheat the oven to 350°F.

4. Prepare the rolling surface by lightly dusting a bit more flour. Knead the dough ball a few times until it's soft. Roll out to 8 mm thickness and cut in circles of 3 ½ inches.
5. Spray a muffin or cupcake tin with a generous layer of cooking spray. And place a dough circle at the bottom. Using a toothpick, poke a few holes at the bottom. Fill the individual tins with the custard.
6. Wet your finger slightly in cold water and run along the rim of each tin. Place another dough circle on top, and firmly but gently seal with your fingers.
7. Brush the top with egg wash and bake in the oven for 40 minutes. Remove from the oven and allow to cool. Dust with icing sugar.

Tartufo

Region of Origin: Calabria

Time: 55 minutes

Serving Size: 4 servings

Prep Time: 15 minutes

Cooking Time: 10 minutes

Salted Caramel Sauce Ingredients:

- ½ cup brown sugar
- ¼ cup water
- ⅓ cup double cream
- 1 teaspoon vanilla extract
- ½ teaspoon flaked sea salt

Tartufo Ingredients:

- 1 cup crushed Oreo cookies
- ½ cup dark chocolate, chopped
- 1-pint vanilla gelato
- 4 maraschino cherries
- 4 twigs of fresh mint

Directions for the salted caramel:

1. In a large saucepan, add the sugar and water, and cook on a medium heat setting until golden brown.
2. Remove from the heat and stir in the remaining ingredients. Allow to cool to room temperature.

Directions for the tartufo:

1. Add the crumbled cookies and chocolate into a sealable plastic bag.
2. Using an ice cream scoop, scoop a ball of gelato into the spoon. Poke a hole in the middle and insert 1 cherry. Cover the hole and gently drop the ball into the bag to cover it with the cookies and chocolate. Place on a tray when done.
3. Repeat the process with the other 3 balls. Freeze for at least 30 minutes.
4. Serve by halving the tartufo and spooning the warm salted caramel on top. Garnish with mint.

Caragnoli

Region of Origin: Molise

Time: 1 hour, 5 minutes

Serving Size: 24 servings

Prep Time: 45 minutes

Cooking Time: 20 minutes

Ingredients:

- 3 free-range eggs at room temperature
- 3 tablespoons brown sugar
- 3 tablespoons canola oil
- 2 cups all-purpose flour
- ¼ teaspoon baking powder
- 1 ½ cup of honey
- 3 cups peanut oil

Directions:

1. In a medium mixing bowl, crack the eggs and beat until frothy. Add the sugar and whisk again. Add the canola oil and whisk well.
2. Combine the flour and dough and sift bits of baking powder into the mixture. Add the dry ingredients to the wet ingredients. Knead the dough for 5 minutes. Cover the bowl with plastic wrap and allow it to rest for half an hour.
3. Cut the dough into 4 equal parts. Roll out in an elongated shape of ⅛ inch in thickness. Form them

into the desired shape. Heat the peanut oil and fry each piece of dough for 30 seconds on a side.

4. Remove the pastry from the oil and place on a tray to drain on the kitchen towel. Heat the honey and drizzle the pastries. Serve immediately.

Conclusion

There are many interesting facts and stories that relate to Italian food and the customs that accompany them.

The 10 top-rated Italian food customs are:

Mealtimes. Italians are very punctual when it comes to the times that they eat their food. Lunch is typically served at one o'clock in the afternoon, and dinner is served at eight o'clock.

Order of events. Traditionally the formal Italian sit-down meal consists of five courses. The sequence is:

1. Antipasto
2. Primo
3. Secondo
4. Contorno
5. Dolce

Lots of dishes to wash. Not everything you see in a movie is real. But in this case, it is. There are always mountains of dirty dishes that need to be washed after every meal. This is because it is a tradition to eat each meal on its own plate.

Salad sides. Salads are served as accompanying dishes, and only a tourist will order this as a dish on its own. Don't feel offended if your request is not adhered to, though.

Cheese and fruit. Each meal is ended with fruit and cheese unique to the region the meal is consumed in.

Coffee. Coffee is nearly close to a religion in Italy and is consumed daily at intervals and anytime in between.

Milk consumption. Milky drinks or consuming milk on its own is reserved for breakfast times only and will be frowned upon otherwise.

Drinks during meals. Wine, mineral water, beer, and soda (kids) are on the list of approved drinks during mealtimes.

Seafood does not get any cheese. No authentic Italian dish will have any form of cheese in it. The fish species all present a delicate palate and will be ruined by the pungent nose of cheese.

Soffritto **- the staple.** The base ingredient in most classic Italian dishes is called *soffrito*. It can be made by combining onion, celery, and carrots that have all been diced finely and frying them in olive oil until fragrant (5 minutes).

Italian Cooking A Glossary of Terms

Arrosto: Meaning any food that is roasted.

Arrosto Morto: Any food that is cooked by roasting it in a pan. This is a term used to describe a method that combines both wet and dry cooking.

All'agro: A green or other ingredient that is cooked briefly then drizzled with olive oil and lemon juice. The lemon juice is also sometimes substituted with vinegar, but less often.

Alla brace: It means to grill.

Al dente: This is the nirvana of pasta when it is perfectly cooked. It should have a firm but elastic texture in your mouth.

Al forno: This means a dish that is cooked in the oven.

Alla griglia: This refers to meat, vegetables, and anything in between that has been barbecued.

Al vapore: Means a dish that is steamed.

Aromi: A collective noun used to describe fragrant herbs such as ginger and garlic.

Antipasto: Translated to English, it means "before the meal" and is referring to the hors d'oeuvre.

Battuto: Refers to vegetables that are finely chopped.

Bianco or in bianco: Bianco or in bianco means white. This can be a pasta or pizza dish that is only made with cheese. Or a lasagne drenched in bechamel sauce.

Bollito: Means boiled when translated into English.

Condimento: Means a dish whereby one ingredient is used as a buddy to flavor another.

Contorno: A dish made of vegetables that is served with the third course of a traditional meal (secondo).

Crema: Refers to a soup created making veggies that were puréed first.

Cucina povera: Refers to a dish that was made from ingredients from a region that is considered to be poor and having little money.

Fare la scarpetta: Means to sop up the sauce and juices in your plate, using slices of bread to mop it up.

Fritto: Referred to as frying a dish. This can be poultry, meat, fish, or even vegetables.

Gnocchi: The Italian word for dumpling.

In umido: A dish that is served with an accompanying tomato-based sauce.

In brodo: Translated, this means "in broth." It is one of the ways to serve pasta, which is a contrast to "dry" pasta.

In padella: Means to fry leafy green vegetables.

Insaporire: An important Italian cooking term, meaning to fry in a base sauce called a sofrito.

In zimino: A term that describes a Tuscan cooking method where the seafood is cooked with leafy greens.

Mantecare: This term refers to whisking, beating, etc. when a sauce or a dish needs to have a smooth, creamy texture.

Minestra: The generic Italian word for soup.

Minestrone: A literal translation meaning "big soup." This is usually a soup that comprises a lot of ingredients that yields into a thick soup.

Odori: This refers to the veggies and herbs that are combined in a *battuto*.

Pasta asciutta: Means a dry pasta that is dressed with sauce.

Pasta all'uovo: Means a fresh egg pasta.

Pasta fresca: Fresh homemade pasta from Italy's Northern region.

Peperoncino: A little red hot chili pepper. It is predominantly used when cooking dishes from Southern Italy.

Primo piatto or primo: Means the first course of a daily Italian mealtime.

Piatto unico: a Meal that is served either during the first or second courses of a meal.

Quanto basta, or q.b: Its literal translation means "more or less."

Ragù: Means a tomato-based sauce that simmers for a prolonged period of time.

Rosolare: Means to lightly fry in oil or butter.

Secondo piatto or secondo: Refers to course number two during a formal sit-down feast.

Spaghettata: A meal that was spontaneously and made unplanned with pasta.

Spianatoia: The wooden surface on which fresh pasta is prepared.

Stuzzichini: Refers to eats or snacks at an event to nibble on.

Sugo: This is a tomato-based pasta sauce.

Trifolati: Means to fry mushrooms.

Un filo d'olio: Means a steady stream of olive oil being poured into a dish.

Vellutata: A soup that has a creamy texture and is made from vegetables.

Zuppa: Means a rustic Italian soup.

Italian Folk Sayings Translated

Chi se move mangia e chi sta fermo secca.

He who moves eats, he who stands still, dries up.

Mangiare per vivere e non vivere per mangiare.

Eat to live and not live to eat.

A tavola non si invecchia.

At the table with good friends and family, you do not become old.

L'Appetito vien mangiando.

Appetite comes with eating.

Chi va a letto senza cena tutta la notte si dimena.

He who goes to bed without eating will regret it throughout the night.

Il riposo da ristoro—solo dopo un buon lavoro.

The rest from refreshment—only after good work. (Meaning) The pleasure one derives from refreshments is enhanced after one has done a good day's work.

Nessuno conosce che cosa sta cucinando nella vaschetta meglio di chi fa la mescolatura.

No one knows what is cooking in the pan better than the one doing the stirring.

Chi la sera i pasti gli ha fatti, sta a gli altri a lavar i piatti.

If one cooks the meal, then the others wash up.

Troppi cuochi guastano la cucina.

Too many cooks spoil the broth.

Chi la vuole cotta e chi la vuole cruda.

Some want it cooked, and some like it raw. (Equivalent) Different strokes for different folks.

La cucina piccola fal la casa grande.

A small kitchen makes the house significant. (Equivalent) The best things in life are free.

Quando la pera e matura, casca da se.

When the pear is matured, it will fall by itself. (Equivalent) All things happen in their own good time.

Una cassetta di mele e arance.

It doesn't make sense to compare two situations to make a point, as the two cases are entirely different from each other.

I frutti proibiti sono i piu dolci.

Forbidden fruit is sweetest.

Esse nufesso qui dice male di macaroni.

One has to be an idiot to speak ill of macaroni.

Amicizie e maccheroni, sono meglio caldi.

Friendships and macaroni are best when they are warm.

Che mangiamo oggi?

What are we going to eat today?

Pane, pesce fritto e baccala!

Bread, fried fish, and dried cod. (Equivalent) There's nothing much to eat.

Chi dorme non piglia pesci.

The early bird catches the worm.

Non si fanno frittate senza rompere le uova.

You have to take action if you want to bring about change.

E meglio l'uovo oggi di una gallina domani.

A bird in the hand is worth two in the bush.
Camminare sulle uova.

Walking on eggshells.

La gallina vecchia fa buon brodo.

The old hen makes a good broth.

Pan di sudore, miglior sapore.

The bread that comes out of sweat tastes better.

Non si vive di solo pane.

One does not live by bread alone.

A chi trascura il poco manchera pane e fuoco.

Stop and smell the roses. Or, Be grateful for what you have.

Pane al pane, vino al vino.

Bread is bread; wine is wine. (Equivalent) To call a spade a spade.

A chi ha fame e buono ogni pane.

All bread is good when you're hungry.

Il pane apre tutte le bocche.

Bread opens all mouths.

E buono come il pane.

English: (Literally) It's as good as bread.

La fame muta le fave in mandorle.

(Literally) Hunger softens fava beans [and makes them sweet]. Meaning: When you're hungry, you don't care about the quality of the food you're eating

Tutto fumo e niente arrosto.

All smoke and no roast. (Meaning): It's no big deal.

Tanto va la gatta al lardo che ci lascia lo zampino.

The cat goes so often to the lard that she will eventually leave her paw print on it.

Belle parole non pascono i gatti.

The poor don't need speeches; they need food.

O di paglia o di fieno purche il corpo sia pieno.

Something is better than nothing.

Aprile freddolino, molto pane e meno vino.

April is a little cold, with lots of bread and not much wine.

Se maggio e scuro, pane sicuro.

If May is dark, bread for sure. (Meaning) If there is poor weather in May, all there will be to eat is bread and not much else.

Bere acqua la mattina e una buona medicina.

Drinking water in the morning is good medicine.

L'acqua corrente non si corrompe mai.

The best things in life are free.

Perdersi in un bicchier d'acqua.

(Literally) To lose oneself in a glass of water. (Equivalent) To make a mountain out of a molehill.

Tanta va la gatta al lardo che ci lascia lo zampino.

(Literally) The pitcher goes so far from the [water] well that it leaves its handle. (Equivalent) A pitcher that is often used is likely to get broken.

Acqua passata non macina piu.

(Literally) Used water doesn't mill anymore. Or Water that's flowed past the mill grinds no more. (Equivalent) What's done, is done. Or It's no use crying over spilled milk.

Una cena senza vino e come un giorno senza sole.

A meal without wine is like a day without sunshine.

Amici e vini sono meglio vecchie.

Friends and wine are best aged.

L'acqua fa male e il vino fa cantare.

Water hurts, and wine makes you sing.

Riempi il bicchere quando e vuoto, vuota il bicchiere quando e pieno, non lo lasciar mai vuoto, non la lasciar mai pieno.

(Literally) Fill your glass when it is empty, empty it when it is full, never leave it blank, never leave it whole.

Luva cattiva non fa buon vino!

Rotten grapes can't give you good wine.

Botte buona fa buon vino.

A good cask makes good wine.

(Dialect): Dumandig' a l'ost' se el gha del bun' vin. El te dis' si!.

(Literally) Ask the innkeeper if the wine is good. Of course, he'll answer yes. Equivalent: Ask a stupid question, and you'll get a silly answer.

Non domandare all'oste se ha buon vino.

Don't ask the host if he has good wine.

Il vino e buono se l'ostessa e bella.

Wine is good if the landlady is beautiful.

Il bicchiere della staffa.

(Literally) The (wine) glass of the stirrup. (Equivalent) One for the road.

Nel vino la verita.

In wine, the truth.

A marzo taglia e pota, se non vuoi la botte vuota

(Literally) In March, cut and prune if you don't want to get hit with nothing. (Equivalent) In March, cut and prune, or you'll not have a good harvest.

References

4 Most Popular Italian Beefs. (2020, November 15). Www.Tasteatlas.com. https://www.tasteatlas.com/most-popular-beefs-in-italy

Animal husbandry - Italy - import, farming. (n.d.). Www.Nationsencyclopedia.com. https://www.nationsencyclopedia.com/Europe/Italy-ANIMAL-HUSBANDRY.html

Appetit, B. (2004, August 20). *Risotto Primavera*. Epicurious. https://www.epicurious.com/recipes/food/views/risotto-primavera-107905

Avey, T. (2012, July 26). *Uncover the History of Pasta | The History Kitchen | PBS Food*. PBS Food. https://www.pbs.org/food/the-history-kitchen/uncover-the-history-of-pasta/

Bagna Cauda. (2004, August 20). Epicurious. https://www.epicurious.com/recipes/food/views/bagna-cauda-2827

BBC Good Food. (n.d.). *A guide to the pasta shapes of Italy*. BBC Good Food. Retrieved November 14, 2020, from https://www.bbcgoodfood.com/howto/guide/guide-pasta-shapes-italy

Boitano, B. (n.d.). *Tartufo*. Food Network. https://www.foodnetwork.com/recipes/brian-boitano/tartufo-recipe-1918820

Button, J. (2020, June 10). *Italian wine labels: Understanding DOCG, DOC & IGT.* Decanter. https://www.decanter.com/learn/italian-wine-labels-understanding-docg-doc-igt-439719/

Capo. (2017, July 18). *spaghetti alla marchigiana.* Iloveitalianfood. http://www.iloveitalianfood.it/en/spaghetti-alla-marchigiana-en/

Casella, C. (2000, October). *Bucatini all'Amatriciana Recipe.* Food & Wine. https://www.foodandwine.com/recipes/bucatini-allamatriciana

Clark, M. (2019, January 24). *Homemade Pasta Dough.* Leite's Culinaria. https://leitesculinaria.com/40229/recipes-homemade-pasta-dough.html

CookiesandKate. (2020, September 30). *Pasta alla Norma Recipe.* Cookie and Kate. https://cookieandkate.com/pasta-alla-norma-recipe/

Costardi Brothers. (n.d.-a). *Veal Tongue Risotto Recipe - Great Italian Chefs. Www.Greatitalianchefs.com.* https://www.greatitalianchefs.com/recipes/piedmont ese-veal-tongue-risotto-recipe

Cottonbro. (2020). None. In *Italian Grandma.* https://www.pexels.com/photo/food-woman-texture-pasta-4057692/

DeLallo. (n.d.). *Italian Tradition: Antipasti | Appetizer or Meal.* DeLallo. https://www.delallo.com/blog/antipasti-meal-social-gathering-or-both/

Eataly. (2019, December 4). *The Origin of the Feast of the Seven Fishes*. Eataly. https://www.eataly.com/us_en/magazine/culture/origin-feast-seven-fishes/ Ehlers, M. (2020). Bread on White Plastic Pack. In *Ciabatta Bread*. https://www.pexels.com/photo/bread-food-wood-breakfast-4198359/

Elda Rita Tessadori. (2013, January 30). *Italian Food Customs and Traditions - Ciao Pittsburgh*. Ciao Pittsburgh. https://www.ciaopittsburgh.com/italian-food-customs-and-traditions/

Essential Italy. (2019a). *10 Interesting Facts About Abruzzo | Essential Italy*. Essential Italy. https://www.essentialitaly.co.uk/blog/10-interesting-facts-abruzzo

Essential Italy. (2019b, January 28). *10 Fun Facts You Didn't Know About Puglia*. Essential Italy. https://www.essentialitaly.co.uk/blog/10-things-didnt-know-puglia

Essential Italy. (2019c, September 30). *10 Fascinating Facts about Umbria*. Essential Italy. https://www.essentialitaly.co.uk/blog/10-fascinating-facts-umbria

Fregola Salad With Olives, Orange Zest & Fresh Herbs. (n.d.). Ginodecampo. https://www.ginodacampo.com/recipe/fregola-salad-olives-orange-zest-fresh-herbs/

Glossary of Italian Cooking Terms. (2017, January 13). Memorie Di Angelina. https://memoriediangelina.com/glossary/

Granoro il Primo. (2012). *Granoro.it - How to recognise good quality pasta.* Granoro.It. https://www.granoro.it/en/c/31/the-world-of-granoro/20/high-quality-production/34/how-to-recognise-good-quality-pasta

greatbritishchefs. (n.d.-a). *Erbazzone Recipe - Great Italian Chefs.* Www.Greatitalianchefs.com. https://www.greatitalianchefs.com/recipes/erbazzone-recipe

greatbritishchefs. (n.d.-b). *Fave e Cicoria Recipe – Fava Bean Purée - Great Italian Chefs. Www.Greatitalianchefs.com. https://www.greatitalianchefs.com/recipes/fave-e-cicoria-recipe-fava-bean-dip*

greatbritishchefs. (n.d.-c). *How to Make Saltimbocca - Great Italian Chefs.* Www.Greatitalianchefs.com. Retrieved November 16, 2020, from https://www.greatitalianchefs.com/how-to-cook/how-to-make-saltimbocca

greatbritishchefs. (n.d.-d). *Parma Ham Parcels Recipe - Great Italian Chefs. Www.Greatitalianchefs.com. https://www.greatitalianchefs.com/recipes/prosciutto-di-parma-parcels-recipe*

greatbritishchefs. (n.d.-e). *Rafanata – Horseradish and Pecorino Frittata Recipe - Great Italian Chefs.*

Www.Greatitalianchefs.com. *https://www.greatitalianchefs.com/recipes/rafanata-recipe*

Gross, T. (2011, March 24). *How "Italian Food" Became A Global Sensation | WBUR News. Wbur.org; WBUR.* *https://www.wbur.org/npr/134628158/how-italian-food-became-a-global-sensation*

Guerero, A. (2020). Cannoli with Pistachios. In *Cannoli.* https://www.pexels.com/photo/cannoli-with-pistachios-4078183/

Guerrero, A. (2020). Lasagna on White Ceramic Plate. In *Lasagna.* https://www.pexels.com/photo/lasagna-on-white-ceramic-plate-4079520/

Horizon Content. (n.d.). Cooked Food on White Ceramic Plate. In *Seafood risotto.* https://www.pexels.com/photo/cooked-food-on-white-ceramic-plate-3763826/

Italian Bread Facts and Nutritional Value. (n.d.). Health Benefits Times. Retrieved November 17, *2020,* from https://www.healthbenefitstimes.com/italian-bread/

Italian Made. (n.d.). *Protected and Certified Italian Products.* Www.Italianmade.com.Au. https://www.italianmade.com.au/page/italian-products

Italian Notes. (2013, March 6). *Gondola facts - 10 interesting facts about Venetian gondolas.* Italian Notes. https://italiannotes.com/gondola-facts/

Italian Word of the Day: Nonna. (n.d.). ThoughtCo. https://www.thoughtco.com/italian-word-of-the-day-nonna-4039731

Italiaoutdoors. (2016, September 22). *Torta Con Le Mele - Apple Cake from Northern Italy.* Honest Cooking. https://honestcooking.com/torta-con-le-mele-apple-cake-northern-italy/

Italy - Agriculture, forestry, and fishing. (2019). In *Encyclopædia Britannica.* https://www.britannica.com/place/Italy/Agriculture-forestry-and-fishing

Italy - Finance. (n.d.). Encyclopedia Britannica. https://www.britannica.com/place/Italy/Finance

Italy hunting trips. (n.d.). Www.Bookyourhunt.com. https://www.bookyourhunt.com/en/hunting-in-italy

Jacqui. (2020a, July 5). *Lasagna Valdostana from the Aosta Valley.* The Pasta Project. https://www.the-pasta-project.com/lasagna-valdostana-from-the-aosta-valley/

zi Lopez Alt, J. (2020, April 7). *Classic Panzanella Salad (Tuscan-Style Tomato-and-Bread Salad) Recipe. Www.Seriouseats.com. https://www.seriouseats.com/recipes/2015/09/classic-panzanella-salad-recipe.html*

Kevmrc. (2020b, March 22). *30 Interesting Facts About Sardinia, Italy - [100% true facts].* Kevmrc.com.

https://www.kevmrc.com/interesting-facts-about-sardinia-italy

Knowles, E., Featherby, L., & Storey, A. (2012, April 9). *Smacafam.* Gourmet Traveller. https://www.gourmettraveller.com.au/recipes/browse -all/smacafam-11447

Knutson, A. (2019, September 24). *Samin Nosrat's Ligurian Focaccia Is Just as Magical as It* Looks. Kitchn. https://www.thekitchn.com/samin-nosrat-salt-fat-acid-heat-ligurian-focaccia-22949343

Kolt, K. (2019, June 12). *Wines of Southern Italy tend to be ripe, round, and juicy, thanks to the weather. The Georgia* Straight. *https://www.straight.com/food/1253841/wines-southern-italy-tend-be-ripe-round-and-juicy-thanks-weather*

LauraLee. (2019a, October 1). *Calabria Italy – 10 Fun Facts.* Digging Up Roots in the Boot. https://digginguprootsintheboot.com/calabria-italy-10-fun-facts/

LauraLee. (2019b, November 26). *Campania Italy-10 Fun Facts.* Digging Up Roots In The Boot. https://digginguprootsintheboot.com/campania-italy-10-fun-facts/

LauraLee. (2020c, February 25). *Friuli Venezia Giulia Italy – 10 Fun Facts.* Digging Up Roots in the Boot. https://digginguprootsintheboot.com/friuli-venezia-giulia-italy-10-fun-facts/

LauraLee. (2020d, March 10). *Molise Italy - 10 Fun Facts.* Digging Up Roots in the Boot. https://digginguprootsintheboot.com/molise-italy-10-fun-facts/

LauraLee. (2020e, March 24). *Tuscany Italy - 10 Fun Facts.* Digging Up Roots in the Boot. https://digginguprootsintheboot.com/tuscany-italy-10-fun-facts/

LauraLee. (2020f, July 7). *Marche Italy 10 Fun Facts.* Digging Up Roots in the Boot. https://digginguprootsintheboot.com/marche-italy-10-fun-facts/

LauraLee. (2020g, August 11). *Valle d'Aosta Italy 10 Fun Facts.* Digging Up Roots in the Boot. https://digginguprootsintheboot.com/valle-daosta-italy-10-fun-facts/

LauraLee. (2020h, September 8). *Emilia Romagna Italy 10 Fun Facts.* Digging Up Roots in the Boot. https://digginguprootsintheboot.com/emilia-romagna-italy-10-fun-facts/

LauraLee. (2020i, October 13). *Lombardia Italy 10 Fun Facts.* Digging Up Roots in the Boot. https://digginguprootsintheboot.com/lombardia-italy-10-fun-facts/

Lazzaris, S. (2019, July 18). *How Rice Is Grown In Italy.* Www.Foodunfolded.com.

https://www.foodunfolded.com/how-it-works/rice-the-italian-way

Lisa. (n.d.-b). *cjarsons Archives*. Very EATalian. Retrieved November 15, 2020, from http://www.veryeatalian.com/tag/cjarsons/

Lovegood, L. (2020). Sliced Bread With Sliced Vegetables on Brown Wooden Chopping Board. In *Italian Antipasti*. https://www.pexels.com/photo/sliced-bread-with-sliced-vegetables-on-brown-wooden-chopping-board-4087611/

Maria. (2018a, December 20). *Caragnoli di Maria: A Molisan Christmas Tradition*. She Loves Biscotti. https://www.shelovesbiscotti.com/caragnoli/

Meat, Poultry and Salumi. (2012, May 21). Living a Life in Colour. https://www.livingalifeincolour.com/kitchen/ingredients/meat-poultry-and-salumi/#go-beef

Miquel, J. (2015, February 4). *Italian Wine & Cheese Pairing Part 2*. Social Vignerons. http://socialvignerons.com/2015/02/04/italian-wine-and-cheese-pairing-part-2/

Nadia. (2019, January 12). *Sicilian Cannoli with Ricotta Filling*. Mangia Bedda. https://www.mangiabedda.com/sicilian-cannoli-with-ricotta-filling/

Necchio, V. (n.d.-a). *Peperoni all'Acciuga Recipe - Great Italian Chefs*. Www.Greatitalianchefs.com https://www.greatitalianchefs.com/recipes/peperoni-all-acciuga-recipe

Necchio, V. (n.d.-b). *Taralli Pugliesi Recipe - Great Italian Chefs.* Www.Greatitalianchefs.com. Retrieved November 14, 2020, from https://www.greatitalianchefs.com/recipes/taralli-pugliesi-recipe

Paola. (2014, March 12). *Gnocchi di Pane Raffermo (Italian Bread Dumplings).* Passion and Cooking. http://www.passionandcooking.com/2014/03/12/gnocchi-di-pane-stale-bread-dumplings/

Pezzaioli, F. (n.d.-a). *Garden snails Brescia (Lumache alla bresciana).* Www.Italyum.com. https://www.italyum.com/specials/172-garden-snails-brescia-lumache-alla-bresciana.html

Pezzaioli, F. (n.d.-b). *Seafood risotto (Risotto alla pescatora).* Www.Italyum.com. https://www.italyum.com/risotto-recipes/183-seafood-risotto8.html

Pixaby. (n.d.). Ribbon Pastry Pasta on Fettuccini. In *Italian Pasta.* https://www.pexels.com/photo/yellow-pasta-spaghetti-eat-42326/

Prestia, T. (2020, August 20). *Pampanella Molisana.* Tinas Table. https://www.tinastable.com/pampanella-molisana/

PRWEB UK. (2017, October 3). *Parma Ham Shares Wine Pairing Ideas.* Benzinga. https://www.benzinga.com/pressreleases/17/10/p10129579/parma-ham-shares-wine-pairing-ideas

Quintanilla, V. (2020, April 19). *Eggplant Parmesan Stacks recipe with wine pairing*. Girl's Gotta Drink. https://girlsgottadrink.com/eggplant-parmesan-stacks-recipe-with-wine-pairing/

Rebecca. (2019, October 4). *13 Great Films set in Sicily to Inspire you to Visit*. Almost Ginger. https://almostginger.com/films-set-in-sicily/

Ricetta Risotto ai mirtilli e speck. (n.d.). Il Cucchiaio d'Argento. https://www.cucchiaio.it/ricetta/ricetta-risotto-mirtilli-speck/

Rosemary. (2018b, November 27). *Easy No Knead Homemade Italian Ciabatta Bread*. An Italian in My Kitchen. https://anitalianinmykitchen.com/homemade-italian-ciabatta-bread/

Rosemary. (2019c, May 13). *Pasticciotti Italian Cream Filled Tarts*. An Italian in My Kitchen. https://anitalianinmykitchen.com/italian-cream-filled-pastry/

roughguides. (n.d.). *Trentino-Alto Adige | Italy Travel Guide | Rough Guides*. Www.Roughguides.com. https://www.roughguides.com/italy/trentino-alto-adige/

Russock, C. (2011, August 23). *Anellini alla Pecorara Recipe | Cook the Book*. Www.Seriouseats.com. https://www.seriouseats.com/recipes/2011/08/anellini-alla-pecorara-recipe.html

Sauced & Found. (n.d.). *Twenty Italian Pantry Staples*. Sauced & Found. Retrieved November 13, 2020, from https://www.saucedandfound.com/blog/2020/5/20/20-italian-pantry-staples

Siano, P. (2014, May 8). *10 Things About Basilicata: It's Not Just a Bunch of Rocks!* Tour Italy Now. https://www.touritalynow.com/blog-basilicata-not-just-a-bunch-of-rocks

Smyth, D. (2019, March 15). *6 Italian Ham Types | eHow.com*. EHow.com. https://www.ehow.com/list_7450792_italian-ham-types.html

Sonoma, W. (2017, October 3). *Easy Seafood Fregola Recipe | Williams Sonoma Taste*. Williams-Sonoma Taste. https://blog.williams-sonoma.com/easy-seafood-fregola-recipe/

Taste Atlas. (n.d.). *Abruzzese Food Homepage: Discover Abruzzese Cuisine | TasteAtlas*. Www.Tasteatlas.com. https://www.tasteatlas.com/abruzzo

The Proud Italian. (2020a, August 2). *Your Favorite Italian Antipasti*. The Proud Italian. https://theprouditalian.com/your-favorite-italian-antipasti/

The Proud Italian. (2020b, September 9). *What Are The 5 Regions of Italy?* The Proud Italian. https://theprouditalian.com/what-are-the-5-regions-of-italy/

Vacayholics. (2011, June 18). *Facts About Piedmont*. Vacayholics. https://vacayholics.com/facts-about-piedmont

van Heerden, F. (2017). Assorted Colour Houses Beside Body of Water. In *Italy Boot*.

Velouria. (2007, May 8). *Goulash Triestino Recipe - Food.com.* Www.Food.com. https://www.food.com/recipe/goulash-triestino-244505

Walks of Italy. (2012, June 8). *8 Things to Love About Emilia Romagna, Italy.* Walks of Italy. https://www.walksofitaly.com/blog/things-to-do/why-visit-emilia-romagna-and-bologna-italy

Walks of Italy. (2019, July 9). *The Regions of Italy.* Walks of Italy Blog. https://www.walksofitaly.com/blog/travel-tips/italy-by-region

Wei-Duan, W. (2017, June 11). *Crescia sfogliata (flaky flatbread) – Le Marche.* Living a Life in Colour. http://www.livingalifeincolour.com/recipes/crescia-sfogliata-flakey-flatbread-le-marche/

World Strides. (2016, October 20). *WorldStrides.* WorldStrides. https://worldstrides.com/blog/2016/10/12-interesting-facts-about-rome/